AROMATHERAPY

WORKBOOK

AROMATHERAPY WORKBOOK

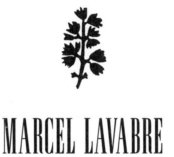

MARCEL LAVABRE

Healings Arts Press
Rochester, Vermont

Healing Arts Press
One Park Street
Rochester, Vermont 05767
www.InnerTraditions.com

Note to the reader: This book is intended as an informational guide. The remedies, approaches, and techniques described herein are meant to supplement, and not to be a substitute for, professional medical care or treatment. They should not be used to treat a serious ailment without prior consultation with a qualified healthcare professional.

Library of Congress Cataloging-in-Publication Data
Lavabre, Marcel
    Aromatherapy workbook / Marcel Lavabre.
        p. cm.
    ISBN 0-89281-346-6
    1. Aromatherapy.   I. Title.
    RM666.A68L38   1990
615'.321—dc20   89–19869
                                                                                CIP

Printed and bound in the Canada

10   9   8   7   6   5   4   3

Text design by Virginia L. Scott
This book was typeset in Caslon with Helvetica Narrow also used as a display typeface

Healing Arts Press is a division of Inner Traditions International

To my daughter, Melissa

Contents

Acknowledgments

I thank the following people:

Jean Valnet, one of the main pioneers of aromatherapy who, with his book *The Practice of Aromatherapy*, contributed greatly to the revival of this art.

Robert Tisserand who first spread the word in the English-speaking world.

Especially Henry Viaud, a French distiller from Provence, who was the first to stress the importance of long, low-pressure distillation and the use of pure and natural essential oils from specified botanical origin and chemotypes and who has not always been credited for his contribution to aromatherapy. Viaud tried to distill practically everything that could be distilled. He was the first to produce a few oils that have recently been introduced on the market (such as St. John's wort and meadowsweet). He also revived the therapeutic use of floral waters. I learned a great deal from this wonderful "honête homme," with his amazing and refreshing curiosity and eagerness for new experiments.

All humble producers who provide me with their oils.

Daniel Penoel for his pioneering work in medical aromatherapy.

All those involved in the bettering and beautifying of our planetary village.

All my students throughout the world.

All the practitioners of the aromatic art.

Introduction

Aromatherapy has known tremendous growth since this book was first published in 1990. It has now become a buzzword, used and abused by marketers and manufacturers of all types and credentials. The availability of essential oils and aromatherapy products has increased dramatically through all types of sources and distribution channels, from health food stores to spa and beauty salons or even department stores and pharmacies. Products with aromatherapy claims (but not much more) can be found in the mass market.

Educational material on the subject is also quite widespread, with new books being published almost every month. A wide selection of classes is available, from one-day beginners' classes to two-year graduation programs. With ever increasing media coverage and celebrities swearing by it, aromatherapy is more fashionable than ever.

But aromatherapy is not just a new trend, a new thing to do, as those who are involved in it can testify. In Europe, where it began more than sixty years ago, aromatherapy is practiced by medical doctors, nurses, and other health professionals. It is taught to medical students in France and is used by some English nurses in their hospitals. Extensive clinical research of aromatherapy is under way, mainly in these countries.

When people first hear about aromatherapy they think about fragrance and perfumes, an alluring world of imagination, magic, and fantasy. But aromatherapy consists simply of using essential oils for healing.

Essential oils are volatile oily substances; they are highly concentrated vegetal extracts that contain hormones, vitamins, antibiotics, and antiseptics. In a way, essential oils represent the spirit or soul of the plant. They are the most concentrated form of herbal energy. Many plants produce essential oils, which are contained in tiny droplets between cells and play an important role in the biochemistry of the plants. They are also responsible for the fragrance of the plants.

Essential oils are used in cosmetics and pharmacy as well as in perfumery. Their field of activity is quite wide: from deep therapeutic action to the extreme subtlety of genuine perfumes. In aromatherapy, the essential oils can be taken internally in their pure form, diluted in alcohol, mixed with honey, or in medical preparations. They are used externally in frictions (localized massage), massage, and inhalations. Finally, they are ingredients of numerous cosmetics and perfumes.

Essential oils can have strictly allopathic effects (meaning that they act like regular medicines); more subtle effects, like those of Bach flower remedies of homeopathic preparations; and psychological and spiritual effects, which constitute their most traditional use. They are also powerful antiseptics and antibiotics that are not dangerous for the body. Aromatherapy is thus, in many cases, an excellent alternative to more aggressive therapies.

Essential oils are the "quintessences" of the alchemists. In this sense, they condense the spiritual and vital forces of the plants in a material form; this power acts on the biological level to strengthen the natural defenses of the body and is the medium of a direct human–plant communication on the energetic and spiritual plane.

Aromatherapy can be used on many different levels. Essential oils are extremely versatile materials: they are both medicine and fragrance; they can cure the most severe physical condition and can reach to the depth of our souls.

Before you start reading this book, though, I warn you: once you step into the world of essences, you will be exposed to one of the most delightful and harmless forms of addiction. Chances are that you will want to know more and more about this amazing healing art. If you allow yourself to be touched by the power of these wonderful substances, you will discover a new world that is actually very old—the almost-forgotten world of nature's fragrances. This is a world without words, a world of images, that you explore from the tip of your nose to the center of your brain—a world of subtle surprise and silent ecstasy.

ONE

Aromatics and Perfumes in History

Since the earliest ages of humanity, aromatic fumigations have been used in daily rituals and during religious ceremonies as an expression and a reminder of an all-pervasive sacredness. Fragrance has been seen as a manifestation of divinity on the earth, a connection between human beings and the gods, medium and mediator, emanation of matter and manifestation of spirit.

In a sense, the origins of aromatherapy can be traced back to the origins of humanity. Some anthropologists believe that the appearance of some form of rituals is the defining moment in the emergence of human culture. Since their origins, rituals have always involved fumigations and the burning of aromatic herbs and woods. Rituals were used mostly in healing ceremonies. What a great intuition! By burning aromatic substances, fumigations diffuse essential oils, which have an antiseptic effect, into the air, bringing about physical healing. At the same time, the fragrance acts on a subtle level for psychic and spiritual healing.

AROMATIC MEDICINE IN EGYPT

The origin of aromatherapy is usually attributed to Ancient Egypt and India. I would date it back to the fabulous and mysterious Kingdom of Sheba, located in the part of the world now called Ethiopia. Ethiopia is considered the cradle of humanity, where the most ancient remains of our distant ancestors have been found.

The Kingdom of Sheba, the "land of milk and honey," was a very prosperous country of the high antiquity. In particular, it controlled the production of the very precious frankincense and myrrh and the trade in spices coming by caravan from India and then by boat through the Red Sea. Sheba is the land from where the three magi came to greet the infant

Christ with gifts of gold, frankincense, and myrrh, the three most precious substances of the time.

There is also the fabulous story of the Queen of Sheba. While the Kingdom of Sheba controlled the trade in frankincense and myrrh, the Queen of Sheba was doing a very hefty business with a tiny kingdom called Israel. Located at the outskirts of the known world, Israel was ruled by a king by the name of Solomon, whose fame had reached all the way to Sheba. The Queen was known to be immensely rich and Solomon had promised his God Yahweh to build a temple the like of which had never been seen on the face of the earth. But the tiny kingdom was broke. Solomon sent emissaries to the Queen, trying to borrow some gold from her. The Queen was intrigued. She decided to undertake the perilous journey across the unforgiving desert to meet her client and potential debtor.

The Queen was young and courageous, and her beauty was stunning. Solomon fell desperately in love with her at first sight. Under the spell of the Queen's magnificent beauty, he neglected his wives and concubines, and even the governing of his kingdom. The Queen eventually decided to return to her kingdom, bearing Solomon's child. Solomon never recovered from his lost love and tried to lose himself in debauchery. He also composed the very famous "Song of Songs," one of the most beautiful love poems and erotic poems in human literature.

There is evidence that the Egyptians borrowed some of their religious and political system from the land of Sheba. In Egypt, medicine was inseparable from religion, and healing always took place in both body and mind. The use of perfumes and aromatics was originally a privilege of the Pharaohs and the high priests. The priests developed a very sophisticated pharmacy, using large quantities of aromatics, which were also used for the preparation and preservation of mummies. The Egyptians made extensive use of substances such as myrrh and frankincense, as well as rose and jasmine. These products were so precious that they were traded as currency.

The Egyptians are considered the inventors of western medicine, pharmacy, and cosmetology. Parallel with the development of medicine and pharmacy, they also developed very refined techniques for skin care, creating beauty recipes that have endured to the present day. Aromatics were the major active ingredients in their skin care preparations. Cleopatra, of course, is legendary for her use of cosmetic preparations and perfumes to enhance her beauty and her powers of seduction. When she sailed to greet the Roman Emperor Marc Anthony, the sails of her ship were soaked in jasmine, one of the most aphrodisiac fragrances. Marc Anthony fell so deeply in love with Cleopatra that he gave up his empire to follow her.

Aromatic medicine emerged from the shade of smoky temples in Egypt—the birthplace of medicine, perfumery, and pharmacy—more than six thousand years ago. The precious substances came from all parts of the world, carried by caravan or by boat: cedar from Lebanon; roses from Syria; spikenard, myrrh, frankincense, labdanum, and cinnamon from Babylon, Ethiopia, Somalia, and even Persia and India.

The priest supervised the preparations in the temples, reading the formulas and chanting incantations, while the students mixed the ingredients. Pulverization, maceration, and other operations could continue for months until the right subtle fragrance was obtained for ceremonial use.

But spiritual matters were not the only concern of the Egyptians. They attached the greatest importance to health and hygiene and were thoroughly familiar with the effect of perfumes and aromatic substances on the body and the psyche. Many preparations were used for both their fragrant quality and their healing power. Kephi, for example, a perfume of universal fame, was an antiseptic, a balsamic, and a tranquilizer that could be taken internally.

The Egyptians also practiced the art of massage and were famous specialists in skin care and cosmetology. Their products were renowned all over the civilized world. The Phoenician merchants exported Egyptian unguents, scented oils, creams, and aromatic wines all over the Mediterranean world and the Arabic peninsula and thereby enhanced the fame and wealth of Egypt.

Embalming was one of the main uses of aromatics. Bodies were filled with perfumes, resins, and fragrant preparations after removal of the internal organs. So strong is the antiseptic power of essential oils that the tissues are still well preserved thousands of years later. In the seventeenth century, mummies were sold in Europe, and

doctors distilled them and used them as ingredients in numerous medicines. The use of aromatics spread from Egypt to Israel, Greece, Rome, and the whole Mediterranean world. Every culture and civilization, from the most primitive to the most sophisticated, developed its own practice of perfumery and cosmetics.

India is probably the only place in the world where this tradition was never lost. With over ten thousand years of continuous practice, Ayurvedic medicine is the oldest continuous form of medical practice. The *Vedas*, the most sacred book of India and one of the oldest known books, mentions over seven hundred different products, such as cinnamon, spikenard, coriander, ginger, myrrh, and sandalwood. The *Vedas* codifies the uses of perfumes and aromatics for liturgical and therapeutic purpose.

DISTILLATION AND ALCHEMY

In Europe, the advent of Christianity and the fall of the Roman Empire marked the beginning of a long period of barbarism and a general decline of all knowledge. Revival came from the Arabic countries with the birth of Islam. Intellectual and cultural activity flourished, as did the arts. Arabic civilization attained an unequaled degree of refinement. The philosophers devoted themselves to the old hermetic art of alchemy, whose origin was attributed to the Egyptian god Tehuti. They renewed the use of aromatics in medicine and perfumery and perfected the techniques. The great philosopher Avicenna invented the refrigerated coil, a real break-through in the art of distillation.

Alchemy, which was probably introduced to Europe by the crusaders on their way back from the Holy Land, was primarily a spiritual quest, and the different operations performed by the adept were symbolic of the processes taking place within the alchemist. Distillation was the symbol of purification and the concentration of spiritual forces.

In the alchemist's vision, everything, from sand and stones to plants and people, was made up of a physical body, a soul, and a spirit. In accordance with the basic principle *solve* and *coagula* (dissolve and coagulate), the art of *spagyrie* consisted of dissolving the physical body and condensing the soul and spirit, which had all the curative power, into the quintessences. The material was distilled over and over to remove all impurities, and the final products were highly potent medicines.

With the expansion of this mysterious art, more and more substances were treated for the extraction of essences. These quintessences were the basis of most medicines, and for centuries essential oils remained the only remedies for epidemic diseases.

THE RENAISSANCE, DECLINE, AND REBIRTH

During the Renaissance, the use of essential oils expanded into perfumery and cosmetics. With further progress in the arts of chemistry and distillation, the production of elixirs, balms, scented waters, fragrant oils, and unguents for medicine and skin care flourished. Nicholas Lemery, the personal physician of Louis XIV, described many such preparations in the *Dictionnaire des drogues simples*. Some have survived until now: Melissa water, Arquebuse water, and the famous Cologne water, for instance, are still produced.

The arrival of modern science in the nineteenth century marked the decline of all forms of herbal therapy. The early scientists had a simplistic and somewhat naive vision of the world. When the first alkaloids were discovered, scientists thought it better to keep only the main active principals of the plants and then reproduce them in laboratories. Thus they discovered and reproduced penicillin (from a natural mold growing on bread), aspirin (naturally present in birch, wintergreen, and meadowsweet), antibiotics, and so on.

Without denying the obvious value of many scientific discoveries, we must acknowledge that the narrow vision of the allopathic medical profession has led to some abuses. Microorganisms adapt to antibiotics much faster than does the human body, making antibiotics inefficient as well as dangerous to the body. Corticosteroids have dreadful side effects; hypnotics, antidepressants, and amphetamines are highly addictive; and so on.

THE BIRTH OF MODERN AROMATHERAPY: AROMATHERAPY IN FRANCE

Aromatherapy per se was formally developed in France in the late 1920s and grew into a mainstream movement in Europe. The term itself was coined by a French chemist by the name of René-Maurice Gattefosse. As the story goes, Mr. Gattefosse, who was a chemist working for the perfume industry, burned his hand in an explosion in his laboratory. A vat full of lavender oil was nearby, and he plunged his hand into it. The pain disappeared instantly, and he recovered so fast that he decided to investigate further the healing power of essential oils. Thus was born modern aromatherapy.

I personally experienced the quasi-miraculous effect of lavender oil on burns on several occasions. A few years ago, while cooking asparagus in a pressure cooker, I spilled more than half a gallon of boiling water on my feet and legs. I removed my socks promptly and applied lavender neat on the whole area and continued applying it every ten to fifteen minutes for a few hours. Not only did the pain disappear, but I never blistered or lost skin! Likewise, when my daughter was twelve years old, she fell asleep on the beach on a very hot summer day, with no prior tan to protect her. She had forgotten to use any sunscreen and the Southern California sun was implacable. She came home redder than a lobster. I instantly applied to her face and body an oil that contains lavender, marjoram, and neroli in a base of sweet almond, hazelnut, and vitamin E. I continued applying it every hour for the first evening and then twice a day for a few days. Again, my daughter didn't blister or peel.

Back to the 1920s, the curative power of essential oils was well known at that time, and many essential oils belonged to the European pharmacopoeia (and still do), which means that they are classified as active medical ingredients.

The French emphasized the medical uses of aromatherapy and conducted extensive research on the antiseptic and antibiotic use of essential oils. Aromatherapy is taught in medical schools and is practiced by medical doctors and naturopaths. Dr. Jean Valnet widely contributed to the popularity of aromatherapy in the sixties and seventies. The major figures today are the conservative Drs. Lappraz, Belaiche, and Duraffour on the one hand, who are the defenders of medical orthodoxy, and Pierre Franchomme, a creative but controversial pioneer, who recently struck gold when he was hired by Estée Lauder to create the "Origins" line. A former Franchomme associate, Dr. Daniel Penoel, recently started working on his own to develop his special techniques on the basis of "live embalming," a massage of the body with pure essential oils.

The French have developed the skin care uses of aromatherapy in only the last ten to fifteen years. French estheticians have grown increasingly attracted to aromatherapy, thanks mostly to lines like Decleor. The French in general, even in the skin care area, tend to use much higher dosages and concentrations than do other European practitioners. Preparations with 10 percent essential oils are not unheard of for professional products, resulting in products that must be used with extreme caution by highly trained professionals. Essential oils and aromatherapy products can be found in all health food stores and many pharmacies and have a stable following. Still, aromatherapy in France has never made headlines the way it has in the United States or the United Kingdom.

The European aromatherapy market evolved in various countries along quite different lines, with each country developing one specific area of application. Only now do we see some overlapping of the various approaches.

British aromatherapy began in the 1950s with Marguerite Maury, a French cosmetologist who lived in London and emphasized uses in skin care and massage, with esoteric undertones. She gave British aromatherapy the spiritualist undertones that it still retains.

Today the major figures in the United Kingdom are Robert Tisserand, Patricia Davis, Shirley Price, and Valerie Worwood. Aromatherapy has become extremely popular in the United Kingdom since the late eighties, when it was known that its adepts included Ms. Thatcher and the royal family, from Princess Diana and Fergie to Prince Charles. Aromatherapy is now a well-developed movement in the United Kingdom, expanding in the health fields through nurses; a group of dedicated nurses gives aromatherapy massage to patients in British hospitals.

Aromatherapy is also gaining scientific credentials, especially in the field of psycho-aromatherapy. Warwick University in particular has been investigating the psychological effects of fragrances for quite some time now.

If the French can be somewhat reckless, the British tend to be overly cautious.

Dosages rarely exceed a few drops per ounce. Their list of contra-indications seems to be growing by the day, with no scientific or anecdotal evidence to sustain it. As pointed out by a frustrated aromatherapist in a recent debate on the subject, there is still not one single reported accident involving essential oils in the United Kingdom.

Curiously, the Europeans have yet to really discover the effect of essential oils as fragrances. Americans, on the other hand, tend to see aromatherapy as the use of fragrances for their mood-enhancing effects, which after all is the most obvious effect of essential oils.

AROMATHERAPY IN THE UNITED STATES

Aromatherapy did not exist in any significant way in the United States until the early 1980s. In fact, when I first moved here in 1981, aromatherapy was still virtually unknown. Aroma Véra, Inc., the company that I founded and still head, has been instrumental in popularizing the concept in the United States and is considered the leader as well as the largest genuine aromatherapy company.

The aromatherapy movement in the United States can be separated into two very different approaches: a genuine approach and a mass-market approach. Genuine aromatherapy is education driven and aims at achieving a synthesis of the various approaches of aromatherapy, which have flourished primarily in Europe. This approach is based on the study of essential oils as chemical substances as well as fragrances. It integrates the various effects of essential oils as healing and curative agents for the body with their properties on the energy and mental levels. Genuine aromatherapy aims to develop practical techniques that integrate the various effects of the oils in a synergistic way. It encompasses body care, skin care, and massage and touches every aspect of daily life. It is part of a natural way of life, an *art de vivre*, that integrates body, mind, and spirit and is geared more toward maintaining health more than curing diseases.

Interest in genuine aromatherapy has been growing steadily over the last fifteen years and is now booming exponentially. The spa, massage, and skin care markets, as well as the health food market, are the most receptive to the concept.

Mass marketers are always looking for the next new trend and, with aromatherapy, they are convinced that they have found the buzzword of the nineties. This has given birth to a rather reduced and oversimplified version of aromatherapy, focusing on the uses of fragrances (and not necessarily natural essential oils) for their mood-enhancing properties.

Americans are without a doubt mass-marketing geniuses, but the contribution of Coca Cola and McDonald's to the fine art of cuisine is questionable, to say the least. While aromatherapy is now under the spotlight of the mass media, receiving intense coverage, there is a danger that it might very well be emptied of its substance in the process. However, the media and the public in general are much more sophisticated today than they ever were. We can hope that genuine aromatherapy will take advantage of the momentum created by mass media to promote the real thing. Aroma Véra is trying to do just that: use the mass-market momentum to advance the genuine art and science of the use of essential oils.

TWO

Aromatherapy: A Multilevel Therapy

SCIENTIFIC RESEARCH AND MODERN AROMATHERAPY

Modern aromatherapy was born at the turn of the century with the works of the French chemist R. M. Gattefosse and has since attracted interest in France, Germany, Switzerland, and Italy. Many studies have been conducted by laboratory scientists and by practicing therapists. Most of this research, somewhat constrained by the dominant scientific ideology, almost exclusively concerns the antiseptic and antibiotic powers of essential oils and their allopathic properties.

Since the early 1980s, however, with the work of Dr. Schwartz at Yale University, and of professors Dodd and Van Toller at Warwick University in England, a better understanding of the Mechanisms of olfaction has opened new, exciting avenues for research and experimentation in aromatherapy.

The Antiseptic Power of Essential Oils

After Pasteur, belief in external agents (microbes, spores, viruses) as the cause of diseases became the basic assumption of official medicine. It was natural, in this context, that the first studies of essential oils should concern their antiseptic properties. Koch himself studied the action of turpentine on *Bacillus anthracis* in 1881; in 1887 Chamberland studied the action of the essential oils of oregano, cinnamon, and clove buds. Other studies by Rideal and Walker and Kellner and Kober proposed different methods of measuring the antiseptic power of essential oils in direct contact or in their vaporized states.

The Aromatogram

With the aromatogram, Dr. Maurice Girault went one step further and provided a useful tool for prescription and diagnosis. Girault, a French gynecologist and obstetrician, has studied the effects of essential oils and tinctures (in association with other natural therapies—homeopathy, minerals, etc.) in gynecology for twenty years. The results of his work were published in *Traité de Phytotherapie et d'Aromatherapie*, Volume 3, *Gynecologie* (Belaiche and Girault, 1979).

In the aromatogram, vaginal secretions on a swab are tested against several essential oils to determine which oil is the most efficient against the specific microorganism. This method has been extend to all infectious disease by French aromatherapy doctors Pradal, Belaiche, Andou, and Durrafour. It has the advantage of dealing with real germs coming from real sites in real patients, rather than from laboratories.

VIRTUALLY NO RESISTANCE PHENOMENA

For all their imperfections and limitations, the various methods of analyzing the germicidal power of essential oils have given scientific validation to aromatherapy. The action of essence on microorganisms is now better understood: essences inhibit certain metabolic functions of microorganisms, such as growth and multiplication, eventually destroying them if the inhibition continues.

Even though there is general agreement on the antiseptic power of essential oils, different authors classify them differently by their antigenetic properties. Since essential oils are products of life, their chemical composition depends on so many factors that it is impossible to obtain exactly the same essence twice. Therefore, different analyses will give different results. According to Jean Valnet, microorganisms show no resistance to essential oils. Recent research on the subject suggests that resistance occurs, but to a far lesser degree than to synthetic antibiotics. This makes sense, as essential oils have a more complex structure and moreover are produced by the defense mechanisms of the plant.

The Power of Living Substances

The real interest of essential oils in medicine lies in their action on the site. Even if they could easily and advantageously be replaced by synthetic products for their antiseptic uses, these synthetics would always be awkward in their interaction with the body as a whole, even though synthetics are chemical reconstructions of components naturally occurring in essential oils.

Essential oils have hundreds of chemical components, most of them in very small amounts. We know that certain trace elements are fundamental for life. In the same way, the power of living products lies in the combination of their elements, and their trace components are at least as important as their main components. No synthetic reconstruction can fully replicate a natural product. It is thus very important to always use natural essential oils.

A HOLISTIC PERSPECTIVE

The human body is a whole, and the interactions taking place between the whole, its parts, and the environment are regulated according to a principle of equilibrium called homeostasis. Homeostasis is an autoregulation process that is ensured by substances such as hormones and the secretions of endocrine glands controlled by the corticohypothalamo-hypophyseal complex. Any external or internal aggression brings a compensatory regulation (hyper- or hypofunctioning) and an imbalance that provokes a defense reaction; the ingestion of chemicals often creates such an imbalance. In disease, chemotherapy consists of answering one aggression with another, creating a state of war highly prejudicial to the battleground—the human body!

We depend on plants in every domain—food, energy, and oxygen—and there is between plants and humans a complementary relationship. We are part of the same whole, which is life itself. This is why plants are not aggressive to the body. (Only abuse of plants can be aggressive.)

Hippocrates, the father of occidental medicine, founded his practice on two basic principles: the principles of similarities (treat the same with the same, the poison with the poison) and the principle of oppositions (find antidotes). The latter, quite straightforward in its application, is the basis of modern medicine (allopathy). The former requires intuition and subtlety; it inspired the theory of similarities as formulated by the great alchemist and philosopher Paracelsus in the Middle Ages. It is also the basic principle of homeopathy and anthroposophic medicine.

From observing the morphology of plants and their different characteristics (their taste, their scent, the environment and soil in which they grow, and their overall vibration), Paracelsus could predict their therapeutic indications. Rudolph Steiner and the anthroposophists adopted the same methods. Their findings have been amazingly accurate and have been largely confirmed by scientific research.

Theories of information and genetics, dealing with the issues of order and chaos, give further justification to such an approach. According to these theories, adaptability and mobility in the use of information are among the chief characteristics of life. A living system (a cell, an organism, a colony of insects, a social group) starts with a certain range of potentials that become actual in a feedback process with the environment. Thus, the embryo and the human being develop from a single primordial cell by differentiation. Life, on the other hand, apparently uses universal structures (such as chromosomic or enzymatic structures). Living systems seem able to "borrow" information from other living systems; to some extent, they are able to incorporate alien information.

If the clue to recovery lies within oneself, it should be very beneficial to give the right kind of information to the body. Therefore, close investigation of the role of essential oils in plants will help one to understand their curative power, while the observation of specific plants will tell us about the healing properties of each individual oil.

Essential oils evidently play a key role in the biochemistry of the plants; they are like the hormones contained in small "bags" located between the cells, and they act as regulators and messengers. They catalyze biochemical reactions, protect the plant from parasites and diseases, and play an important role in fertilization. (Orchids, the most fascinating family of plants, have developed this process to a high degree, attracting the most suitable insects to carry precious pollen to their remote sexual partners.)

Essential oils carry information between the cells and are related to the hormonal response of the plant to stressful situations. They are agents of the plant's adaptation to its environment. It is not surprising, then, that they contain hormones. Sage, traditionally known to regulate and promote menstruation, contains estrogen. Ginseng, a well-known tonic and aphrodisiac, contains substances similar to estrone. Estrogens can also be found in parsley, hops, and licorice. Rosemary increases the secretion of bile and facilitates its excretion.

Essential oils control the multiplication and renewal of cells. They have cytophilactic and healing effects on the human body (especially lavender, geranium, garlic, hyssop, and sage). According to Jean Valnet, they have anticarcinogenic properties. They are often present in the outer part of leaves, in the skin of citrus fruits, and in the bark of certain trees. Cosmetic applications are among their oldest uses.

Most aromatic plants grow in dry areas, and the essential oils in them are produced by solar activity. In the anthroposophic vision, essential oils are the manifestation of the cosmic fire forces. They are produced by the plant's cosmic self. In them, matter dissolves into warmth. Therefore, they are indicated for diseases originating in the astral body.

AROMATICS AND THE SOUL

Aromatherapy acts at different levels. There is first an allopathic action due to the chemical composition of the essential oils and their antiseptic, stimulant, calming, antineuralgic, or other properties. There is a more subtle action at the level of information, similar to the action of homeopathic or anthropsophic remedies. Last but not least, essential oils act on the mind. In fact, they are most traditionally used as basic ingredients of perfumes. Generally speaking, pleasant odors have obvious uplifting effects. According to Marguerie Maury in *The Secret of Life and Youth*:

> Of the greatest interest is the effect of fragrances on the psychic and mental state of the individual. Power of perception becomes clearer and more acute, and there is a feeling of having, to a certain extent, outstripped events. ... It might even be said that the emotional trouble which in general obscures our perception is practically suppressed.

Anatomy of Olfaction

Recent research conducted in Europe, the United States, and the former Soviet Union reveals that the effects of odors on the psyche many be more important than scientists have suspected. The University of Warwick, England, has been conducting fascinating research on this subject (see Theimer, *Fragrance Chemistry: The Science of the Sense of Smell*). Figure 1 illustrates the anatomy of olfaction.

The sense of smell acts mostly on a subconscious level; the olfactory nerves are directly connected to the most primitive part of the brain, the limbic system—our connection with our remote saurian ancestors, our distant reptile cousins. In a sense, the olfactory nerve is an extension of the brain itself, which can then be reached directly through the nose. This is the only such open gate to the brain.

The limbic system, originally known as the rhinecephalon ("smell brain"), is the part of the brain that regulates the sensorimotor activity and deals with the primitive drives of sex, hunger, and thirst. Stimulation of the olfactory bulb sends electrical signals to the area of the limbic system concerned with visceral and

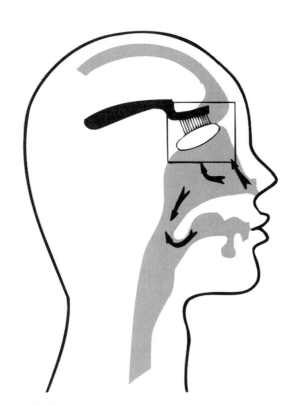

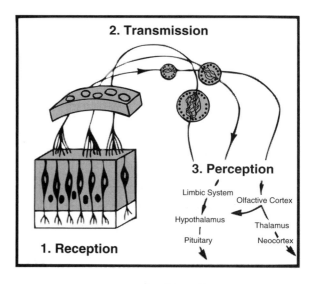

Fig. 1. The Anatomy of Olfaction

behavioral mechanisms; they directly affect the digestive and sexual systems and emotional behavior. In fact, the brain's electrical response to odors is about the same as the one correlated with emotions. (In the French language the same verb, *sentir,* is used for "to smell" and "to feel.") The processes of olfactory reception are largely unconscious; we are mostly unaware of our scent environment. For some yet-unexplained reason, whenever we are in contact with a new odor, we lose our consciousness of it after a while. The electrical signals correlated to this odor still continue to reach the brain, but the contacts with our conscious centers have been shut off. This shows how little control our conscious centers have on the olfactory stimulations.

The sense of smell is very sensitive: we can detect up to one part of fragrant material in 10,000 billion parts or more. A trained nose can differentiate several hundred different odors. However, we have no proper vocabulary to talk about odors. We say that something smells like a rose, strawberry, skunk, or whatever. The olfactory nerves terminate in a part of the brain that does not use the same kind of logic as our intellectual centers. Although odors form a kind of communication system, they cannot be developed as a language; they work through associations and images and are not analytical.

In *Perfumery: The Psychology and Biology of Fragrance* (Van Toller and Dodd, Eds.), E. Douek describes various olfactory abnormalities. According to the author, anosmia, the total inability to smell, is always accompanied by some elements of depression, which can often become severe. With loss of the sense of smell, people also lose the sense of taste. The world becomes dull and colorless.

Even more interesting is parosmia, or olfactory illusion (usually related to a perception of bad odors). In such cases, shy and withdrawn people tend to feel that the unpleasant odors they perceive emanate from themselves, while people with paranoid tendencies perceive them as coming from others. The latter suspect imaginary plots in their associates and generally show tyrannical tendencies. According to Douek, the French King Louis XI suffered from this affliction. He was very good at filling up his prisons and inventing sophisticated tortures to obtain confessions from his victims. It might be instructive to investigate the olfactory sanity of the most prominent tyrants throughout history!

Olfactory System and Sexual Mechanisms

Mammals release sexual olfactory signals called pheromones through specialized scent-producing apocrine glands. In humans, most of these glands are located in the circumanal and anogenital region, the chest and the abdomen, and around the nipples, with some variations between the different races. (According to D. M. Stoddart, pheromone production is minimal among Mongoloids, especially Korean Huanghoids.)

D. M. Stoddart notes in *Perfumery: The Psychology and Biology of Fragrance* (Van Toller and Dodd, Eds.) that most perfumes contain ingredients that mimic these sexual olfactory signals, such as civet, musk, or castoreum, and also substances like sandalwood (remarkably similar, according to the author, to androsterol, a male human pheromone). According to G. H. Dodd, humans secrete musk-like molecules, and therefore we experience this type of odor in utero, which could explain the universal liking for it. The main function of perfumes would then be to heighten and fortify natural odors, rather than to cover them.

The connection between olfaction and the sexual system takes place through the hypothalamic region. According to D. M. Stoddart in *Perfumery: The Psychology and Biology of Fragrance* (Van Toller and Dodd, Eds.),

> The hypothalamic region is a major receiver of olfactory neurones, and releases a variety of . . . hormones which pass to the anterior pituitary via the hypophyseal portal system, and induces the pituitary to secrete the suite of hormones which governs and controls the mammalian sexual cycles.

The synchronization of menstrual periods in girls' boarding schools is a well-known phenomenon. Several studies have shown that such synchronicity could be caused by axillary secretions (i.e., by pheromones).

In another now-famous experiment, set up in a kindergarten, children playing near a pile of T-shirts worn by their mothers could accurately find their own mothers' T-shirts within a very short time. Most

of them would then retire to a corner with the T-shirt and quiet down. Although this experiment is not directly concerned with sexual matters, it shows the strong olfactory component of the mother–infant bond. It is also worth noting that breast-fed babies develop a much stronger olfactory bond to their mother than do bottle-fed ones.

The Gate to the Soul

When Sigmund Freud opened the Pandora's box of the unconscious at the beginning of this century, he suspected sexual drives to be the central feature of the show being played on our private stage. He considered the repression of smell to be a major cause of mental illness and suspected that the nose was related to the sexual organs. (Allergy to odors is a psychosomatic disease.)

If psychoanalysis and its avatars are to explore the unconscious from the mental side, the nose and the sense of smell give access to Pandora's box from the other side: the unknown side, the saurian side, from the origin of ages. The subtle emanations create a diffuse network that connects us to the unconscious of species, and to life itself. The strongest and deepest experiences are often accompanied by olfactory sensations. All traditions, even the most puritan, have known the power of fragrances; every religion knew their ceremonial use (usually in connection with sounds and colors) to generate elation among the faithful. Mystics or visionaries experience heavenly fragrances in their deepest ecstasy. Such people may eventually die in the "odor of sanctity."

Fragrances can bring about the deepest but most fugitive sensations. Like happiness, or love, or laughter, they catch you, almost by surprise, and fade away as soon as you try to grasp them. As you walk along the street, pull out the weeds in your backyard, hike on a trail, or sip your coffee, a mysterious emanation suddenly strikes your nose and the magic unfolds. In an instant of rapture, waves of delight run through your entire body, bringing about images and new sensations. But if you try to analyze what is going on, the experience disappears like a soap bubble; if you try to talk about it, you will soon fall short of words.

According to Jean-Jacques Rousseau, the sense of smell is imagination itself. Some authors needed olfactory sensations to stimulate their creativity. Guy de Maupassant, for instance, used to soak strawberries in a bowl of ether. Schillar filled the top drawer of his desk with ripe apples.

The sense of smell is closely related to memory; olfactory memories are very accurate and almost indelible. A French psychoanalyst, André Virel, used fragrance to bring forth hidden memories. The odor and taste of a madeleine dipped in a cup of tea inspired Marcel Proust to write one of the most remarkably precise and vivid works of introspection, and a masterpiece of literature.

We probably all have our own private madeleines. Syringa, to me, is one of the most heavenly fragrances. It transports me to a space of undisturbed peacefulness where I can vividly recall the vegetable garden of my early childhood, with its fallen trellis, its dry wall above the dirt road leading to the spring, and its basin of fresh running water. There is a huge fig tree in the corner just above the road and stone shed, falling in ruins on the other side with a bush of syringa in the middle. I am leaning against the bush now in full bloom; I have been here for hours. Out there, behind the stone arch, is the farm, and then the world. But here, the warm and gentle sun of May envelops my frail body; the divine fragrance of syringa bathes my soul. I am totally at home. Why should I ever move?

PSYCHOTHERAPY AND AROMATHERAPY: A WIDE OPEN FIELD

Since the olfactory system is such an open gate to the subconscious, one would expect that psychotherapy could benefit from the use of olfactory stimuli for the cure of psychological disorders. Very little research has been done in this area, however, possibly because it is hard to systematize any kind of therapeutic procedure. The sense of smell is very private. Each individual's associations are different. Dr. A. D. Armond, for instance, reported the case of an anxious patient who worked on motor bikes and kept an oily washer in his pocket for comfort in times of stress.

Still, aromatherapy can offer some valuable tools to the practitioner. Oils such as neroli, lavender, marjoram, rose, and ylang-ylang have been traditionally used for their calming effects in stress reduction. Jasmine is a wonderful uplifting oil for the treatment of depression or anxiety, and there are many more (see Chapter 7 and Appendices I and II). Diffusion is probably one of the best methods of using essential oils in this way.

One procedure often used by therapists is to prepare an appropriate blend of oils to use during the therapeutic session. The patient can then use the same blend at home to further the treatment. This method is particularly efficient when used in conjunction with any technique conducive to deep relaxation (such as hypnosis, meditation, yoga, or certain types of massage), as the olfactory stimuli are then more likely to have a deep impact on the patient.

Obviously, psychoaromatherapy (a term coined by Robert Tisserand) is still a wide-open field, where experimentation should be encouraged. With minimal caution, no adverse side effects can be expected from the use of aroma in psychotherapy, while the potential benefits appear to be unlimited. I am personally very curious about any finding in this fascinating domain and invite my therapist readers to share their experience in this area with me.

UN JE NE SAIS QUOI, UN PRESQUE RIEN

Essential oils and fragrances have been extensively used for well-being—one of the main keys to health—since the beginning of civilization. Vladimir Jankelevitch, a French philosopher who gave cooking classes to his delighted students in the venerable Sorbonne, talked about *un je ne sais quoi, un presque rien* ("an I-don't-know-what, an almost-nothing") to characterize the subtle quality of an *art de vivre*, which can be extended to the basic jubilation of just being alive. This *je ne sais quoi*, this *presque rien* that is the mark of genuine art, of elegance, of humor, which differentiates a real meal from a mere quantity of proteins, calories, vitamins, and minerals, describes perfectly the contribution of fragrances to the quality of life. It is unpredictable, it cannot be analyzed by any scientific method, and yet it can be experienced. According to Goethe, the most evolved plants go through a transformation from the primitive germ to the exuberance of the flower in a natural movement toward spirituality where the flower, in its impermanence and openness, represents an instant of rapture and jubilation. Fragrance is a manifestation of this jubilation.

Fragrances have their own language. Better than any word, they can express the most subtle feelings. Much is revealed about a person by his or her choice of fragrance and how that fragrance reacts with the skin. Everyone has his or her specific odor, which changes depending on the physical and mental state of the individual; thus, dogs can find lost people and criminals. Smell may, in fact, be a determinant in the establishment of relationships. It has also been a traditional tool for diagnosis (each disease is said to have its specific odor).

Aromas, even if they cannot change an individual, may help to create a positive groundwork if properly chosen. Fragrances stimulate the dynamic and positive aspect of the being by an effect of resonance. During the Renaissance, the *grande dames* had their own secret perfumes; numerous systems associate perfumes with astrological signs, dominant planets, or morphological characteristics.

In conclusion, even though it can relieve symptoms, aromatherapy primarily aims at curing the causes of diseases. The main therapeutic action of essential oils consists in strengthening the organs and their functions and acting on the defense mechanism of the body. They do not do the job for the body; they help the body do its own job and thus do not weaken the organism. Their action is enhanced by all natural therapies that aim to restore the vitality of the individual. Maurice Girault recommended using them in connection with minerals, homeopathy, and psychotherapy. To this list I add nutrition, as food is the basis of animal life; depending on its quality, food can be the best medicine or the main cause of disease.

THREE

Essential Oils:
Extraction and Adulteration

ESSENTIAL OILS IN THE PLANT

Essential oils are the fragrant principle of the plant. They are the chemical components that give a plant its characteristic fragrance. In the spiritualistic approach to aromatherapy, essential oils are considered the life force, the energy of the plant. Alchemists regard them as the quintessence, the soul, the spirit of the plant. Anthroposophists see them as produced through the action of astral forces in the plant.

Essential oils are a type of vegetal hormone that helps the plant in its adaptation to the environment. From a biochemical point of view, they can be considered part of the plant's immune system. In extreme climates, such as the Arabian desert, certain plants use essential oils as a protection against the sun. Myrrh and frankincense bushes are surrounded by a very thin cloud of essential oils, which filters the sun's rays and freshens the air

around the bushes. *Dictamus fraxinella,* a plant of the same family that grows in the Sinai, is so literally endowed with resinous oil glands that the resinous vapor perpetually surrounding the shrub burns with a brilliant glow when lit. (According to Roy Genders, the burning bush that Moses saw in the Sinai could have been caused by such a phenomenon.) Essential oils also protect the plant from diseases and parasites.

The plant uses essential oils from its flowers for its reproductive process. It attracts specific insects by releasing fragrances that mimic the insect's pheromones to facilitate pollination. In a way, essential oils from flowers are part of the plant's sexual system. We describe many essential oils that have aphrodisiac properties and other properties that relate to reproduction and sexuality (emmenagogues, hormone balancers, PMS or menopause relief, etc.).

Certain essential oils have the power to repel insects that could be harmful to the plant. For example, citronella and geranium are mosquito repellent and lavender and spike repel fleas and mites. They sometimes even act as natural selective weedkillers, creating a territory around their roots where certain other plants cannot grow. Organic and biodynamic farmers know how to take advantage of this phenomenon in their work: certain plants have dynamic effects on the growth of specific plants while inhibiting others.

The plant stores its essential oils in small pouches. It is important to note that plants do not use essential oils in their pure form. Plants store essential oils in specific areas and retrieve them in a diluted form when they are needed for the plant's biochemical processes. Humans, like plants, should not use essential oils in their pure form. Do not try to be smarter than plants!

Essential oils are usually located on the outer part of the plant. They can be seen on the skin of citrus fruits, for instance, or on the surface of the leaves, which act as the skin of the plant. This indicates the strong affinity of essential oils for the skin.

PHYSICAL PROPERTIES OF ESSENTIAL OILS

Essential oils are chemically very different from vegetable oils or other types of fats. Aromatic molecules are much smaller than fatty acids. They are carbonic chains that generally have ten carbons. A few have fifteen carbons, and some rare components go up to twenty carbons.

What characterizes essential oils is the fact that they are volatile, which means that they evaporate completely when exposed to the air. If you put one drop of vegetable oil, such as canola oil, on a piece of paper, it will stain and the stain will remain. If you put a drop of essential oil on the same piece of paper, it will eventually evaporate completely. This volatile quality is what allows us to smell essential oils in the first place. It is also the property that allows us to extract essential oils through distillation.

Essential oils are lypophile, which means that they are readily absorbed by vegetable oils, waxes, and fats. This property allows us to make flower oils and allows the extraction process called enfleurage. The lypophilic property of essential oils is very useful for the preparation of massage oils and facial oils. It also means that essential oils applied externally absorb rapidly into the skin and the underlying tissues thanks to their high fatty content.

Essential oils are hydrophobic; that is, they do not mix with water. This property is necessary for the final stage of steam distillation, in which the essential oils are separated from the water. Hydrophobia makes essential oils difficult to use in water-based products. In general, it is not a good idea to put essential oils into water, as they will float on the surface. Essential oils are partially soluble in alcohol. The amount of an essential oil that can be mixed with alcohol depends on the individual essential oil and on the proof of the alcohol.

The chemistry of essential oils is rather complex. It varies during the day and throughout the year; it depends on the part of the plant being distilled (root, wood, bark, leaf, stem, flower, seed), the variety, the soil, even the climate. The oils are mainly constituted of terpenes, sesquiterpenes, esters, alcohols, phenols, aldehydes, ketones, and organic acids. They contain vitamins, hormones, antibiotics, and/or antiseptics. The yield of essential oils varies between 0.005 and 10 percent of the plant. Thus, 1 pound of essential oil requires 50 pounds of eucalyptus or lavandin, 150 pounds of lavender, 500 pounds of sage, thyme, or rosemary, and 2,000 to 3,000 pounds of rose!

TRADITIONAL METHODS OF EXTRACTION

Oil Infusion

Extraction by fats, also called oil infusion, is probably the oldest method of obtaining essential oils. Oil infusion consists of soaking the plants in vegetable oil in a glass jar and exposing them to the sun for one to two weeks. The plants are then strained out, and more herbs are added to the scented oil. Shepherds and farmers in Provence, in southeast France, prepare the "red oil" by soaking St. John's wort flowers in olive oil for two weeks. This oil has amazing healing properties, especially with burns.

Enfleurage

In enfleurage, another method of extraction, a layer of fresh flowers is placed on an oil-soaked cloth or on a thin layer of lard. The flowers are replaced by fresh ones every day until the right concentration is obtained. Although these different methods do not allow a separation of the essential oils, the products obtained are particularly suited to creams, ointments, liniments, massage oils, and bath oils.

Cold Expression

Some essential oils can be extracted by cold pressure; this process is commonly used for citrus fruits. The outer layer of the fruit peel contains the oil and is removed by scrubbing. Through centrifigation, the oil then separates from the pulp. (If you pinch the peel of a lemon or an orange in front of a candle flame, you can see the oil come out when it burns in the flame.)

The Origin of Distillation

Distillation is still the most common process of extracting essential oils. Historians do not agree on its origin, but most attribute it to Avicenna, the famous Arab philosopher, physician, and alchemist, who lived at the turn of the millennium. However, Zozime, renowned Egyptian chemist living in the third century A.D., wrote about numerous designs of stills adorning the wall of a temple in Memphis. It is quite likely, in fact, that the Egyptians were aware of a primitive process of distillation.

In the first century A.D., Dioscorides already wondered about the origin of distillation. He reported that, according

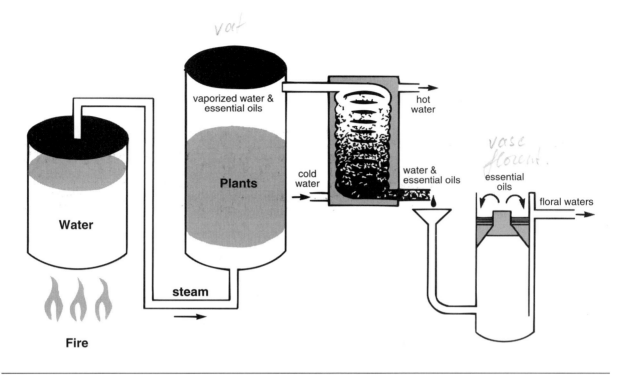

vat

vaporized water &
essential oils

hot
water

Plants

cold
water

water &
essential oils

vase florent.

essential
oils

floral waters

Water

steam

Fire

Fig. 2. The Steam Distillation Process

to oral tradition, a physician baked pears between two dishes. When he took off the upper dish, he noticed that the steam covering it smelled and tasted like a pear. It inspired him to build elaborate instrument for the extraction of the "quintessences" of medicinal plants.

A still consists of a vat: a large cylindrical tank, which contains the plants. Steam is sent through the plants from the bottom of the vat and evaporates the oils. The vat is covered by a special lid (*col de cygne* or swan neck), which collects the steam and sends it to the coil, usually refrigerated with running water, where the steam is condensed. The mixture of condensed water and oil separates naturally by decantation in *vase florentin* (florentine vase). This is illustrated in Figure 2.

Many farms in southeastern France had such equipment until the turn of the century. Since the vats were relatively small (the main vat contained less than 100 gallons), they were often used for extracting essential oils (mostly wild lavender) in the summer and distilling brandy in the winter. Today, wild lavender has almost disappeared and nobody picks it anymore (I bought one of the last batches a few years ago), but there are still many distilleries in Provence. In some areas, every village has at least one. The vats are much larger (some have up to six vats containing over 1,500 gallons), and the water is now heated in a separate boiler. The people there distill mostly lavandin, a hybrid of lavender that gives a better yield of lower-quality essential oil. They also distill true lavender, hyssop, clary sage, and occasionally tarragon or cypress.

Extraction by Solvents

This relatively modern technique is used worldwide for higher yield or to obtain products that cannot be obtained by any other process. The plants are immersed in a suitable solvent (acetone or any petroleum by-product), and the separation is performed chemically by distillation under special temperatures that condense the oil but not the solvents. Unfortunately, such oils always contain some traces of solvent and are therefore not suitable for aromatherapy.

For the fabrication of "concretes" the material is usually soaked in hexane. The mixture is then concentrated by double distillation, and the final product has a creamy consistency due to the presence of residual solvents and waxes from the plants. The "absolutes" are obtained from concretes by dilution in alcohol, double filtration, and double concentration, which eliminates most waxes and residual solvents.

This method is used widely for roses, neroli (orange blossoms), cassia, and tuberoses. It is the only way to extract oils from jasmine, honeysuckle, carnation, and others. Concretes and absolutes are extensively used in cosmetics and perfumery; they should not be used for aromatherapy.

Hypercritical Carbon Dioxide Extraction

Hypercritical carbon dioxide extraction is a new process that has raised great hopes among perfumers and aroma-therapists. How is it hypercritical?

Any substance can exist in three different states: gas, liquid, and solid. Every substance may be in any of these three states depending on its temperature and pressure. In addition, certain substances can be found in the hypercritical state—that is, they are neither liquid nor gas, but rather they are both; they disperse as readily as a gas (i.e., almost instantaneously) and have solvent properties.

Under any given temperature, most substances go from gaseous at low pressure (close to vacuum for heavy substances like metal) and to liquid when the pressure increases. Some substances, though, never become liquid if their temperature is maintained over their hypercritical temperature. They will instead be in the hypercritical state when pressure increases over hypercritical pressure.

Carbon dioxide (a fairly inert gas naturally occurring in the air that we breathe) has the power to become hypercritical. Even better, its hypercritical temperature is 33°C (a little over room temperature). Hypercritical carbon dioxide then becomes an excellent solvent of fragrances and aromatic substances. The advantages are that the whole operation takes place at fairly low temperature, and therefore the fragrance is not affected by heat; the extraction is almost instantaneous (a few minutes) and complete. Because the solvent is virtually inert, there are no chemical reactions between the solvent and the aromatic substances. In comparison, steam distillation requires one to forty-eight hours, it always leaves some residues of essential oils, and many substances are hydrolyzed or oxidized in the process.

Unlike the products of regular solvent extraction (concretes, absolutes, oleoresins), the solvent can be easily and totally removed, just by releasing the pressure. The whole process takes place in a closed chamber, which means that even the most volatile and most fragile fractions of the fragrance can be collected. Consequently, the end product is as close as anyone can get to the plant's aromatic substance.

Hypercritical carbon dioxide extraction then appears to be an aromatherapist's dream come true. Unfortunately, the hypercritical pressure for carbon dioxide is over 200 atmospheres (200 times the regular atmospheric pressure!), requiring very heavy and expensive stainless-steel still equipment.

As far as I know, this process is still in an experimental stage. Pilot units have been built in a few high-tech laboratories in France, Germany, the United States, and Japan. (I visited the French pilot in 1987; its capacity was less than 2 gallons, whereas a regular steam still has a capacity of up to 2,000 gallons.) Only small amounts of hypercritical extracts have been produced so far, but commercial production may not be too far down the line. Such products are likely to remain fairly costly for the time being.

Yield of the Most Common Essential Oils

The yield of essential oils varies greatly from one plant to another. To make one kilogram (kg) of essential oil, it takes about:

20 kg of clove buds
30 kg of eucalyptus leaves
35 kg of lavandin
150 kg of lavender
300 kg of peppermint
300 kg of Moroccan rosemary
500 kg of red thyme
600 kg of French rosemary
800 kg of clary sage
1,000 kg of chamomile
3,000 kg of rose
10,000 kg of melissa

The difference in yields leads to wide variations in price from one essential oil to another. Obviously, eucalyptus oil will be rather inexpensive, while rose oil is going to be very costly.

Floral Waters, Distillates, and Hydrolates

Floral water, distillates, or hydrolates are obtained by sending steam through the plants and condensing this steam; they are often a by-product of distillation, in which case they are recovered from the florentine vase after separation of the essential oils. The best floral waters are obtained by cohobation, a process that continuously recycles the distillate. The amount of water used for distillation is proportional to the quantity of plant; the overflow from the florentine vase is sent back into the boiler, and steam is sent through the plant material until it is saturated.

Hydrolates contain the water-soluble active principles of the plants. They retain a small amount of essential oils (about 0.2 grams per liter) that disperses in an ionized form, so that the product is less likely to cause skin irritation. They were traditionally used for skin care, for the disinfection of wounds, and for healing. Because hydrolates are milder and easier to use than essential oils, their utility in skin care and cosmetics is considerable. Rose flower water, orange blossom water, chamomile water, and bluet water are among the most renowned.

Do It Yourself

All an amateur distiller needs is a pressure cooker. Place the plants on a screen above the water. Replace the valve with a plastic hose (2 to 5 feet long), boil the water, run cold water on the hose, and collect the floral water and oils in any suitable container. You can separate the oils by decantation in glass bottles. You will not, of course, produce large amounts of oils, but their quality will be excellent and you will also obtain plenty of floral water with which to prepare your own cosmetics, creams, and shampoos. I should warn you, however, that distillation is an incurable addiction!

HOW TO KEEP YOUR ESSENTIAL OILS

Essential oils are precious products that can be very expensive. (You will understand why when you start making your own.) Store them in tightly closed dark glass bottles to prevent their deterioration by light or by air. They should also be protected from temperature variations; prolonged heat is not good for them. Under normal conditions, essential oils can be considered fresh for three years after their extraction.

THE QUALITY ISSUE

The quality of the essential oils available on the market has improved substantially since this book's first publication, thanks mostly to better consumer education. Good quality essential oils are now easily available through spas and skin care salons, health food stores, and specialty stores. Although some offer products with aromatherapy claims, the mass market has yet to discover real essential oils.

Quality is still an issue and consumers should be watchful of possible adulterations, which can be natural or synthetic. There are two main reasons for adulterations. The chemical composition of essential oils of a given plant can vary to a large extent, depending on the variety, the time, the soil, the methods of cultivation and distillation. The oil of thyme, for instance, varies from 100 percent thymol to 90 percent carvacrol, with some varieties containing citral or geraniol. In addition, many of the basic components, such as linalol, cineol, borneol, citral, and nerolidol, are present in different essences. Knowing the main components of a given essential oil, it is then possible to reconstitute it using cheaper essential oils or their components. Rose, for instance, is often falsified with geranium, lemongrass, palmarosa, terpenic alcohol, stearine, etc.

Recent advances in chemistry have flooded the market with synthetic essential oils. These synthetic reconstitutions are mostly used in the food or cosmetic industry, but also in perfumery and pharmacy. The chemical substances present in the oils are in perpetual interaction, and the kind of interaction taking place basically depends on the way these substances have been put together. The action of essential oils depends also on the processes taking place in them. Therefore, natural or synthetic reconstitutions will never replace the natural oils. For aromatherapy as well as for perfumery or cosmetics, one should use only the best quality of essential oils.

The oils extracted by cold pressure are of course the closest to the products present in the plant, but only a few oils can be extracted by this method. Steam distillation yields the second best quality. Wild plants growing in unpolluted areas or organic plants of course yield the best quality of oil. Nonorganic products are not recommended, as many synthetic pesticides are soluble in the plants' aromatic substances and might be concentrated in the oil.

Various analytical processes are available for evaluating the quality of an essential oil, the most common being gas chromatography and mass spectrometry. Such methods allow an experienced specialist to detect most adulterations, but will not provide any information on more subtle criteria of quality, such as country of origin or method of growth. Such methods are unpractical for the average consumer who must rely on a trusted supplier.

Finding a reliable supplier is challenging because of the nature of the market: the essential oil market is rather complex and one needs to be very familiar with it to be able to obtain optimum quality. Most of the trade in essential oils is done through brokers, and the major market for essential oils is still the fragrance and the food industries. The aromatherapy market is a growing but still marginal market. The food industry trade concerns a few selected oils, such as citrus, mint, and spices. The widest variety is being used by the fragrance industry. For that industry, consistency in smell and in price is more important than purity. Most fragrance formulations include hundreds of ingredients, some natural, some synthetic. It is very important for the compounder that all ingredients maintain consistency. But nature is not consistent. From one crop to the next, from one origin to the next, the fragrance of an essential oil may vary substantially. Such variations may be buffered by addition of synthetic or natural components. Price may also fluctuate wildly. A given oil may double in price after a natural disaster in an important area of production. For instance, floods in China almost tripled the price of geranium in 1995. Price variations are buffered the same way. This explains why it can be challanging to obtain reliable quality essential oils on the open market.

Here are some guidelines for selecting a supplier of essential oils:

♦ Make sure that your supplier can provide as detailed information as possible about the essential oils they offer: botanical name, country of origin, and, if possible, method of growth.

♦ Price is an indication, but make sure that your supplier does not take advantage of your concern about quality to charge excessive prices: oils such as eucalyptus, especially eucalyptus globulus, or orange, lemon, cedarwood, or pine are plentiful and inexpensive. Rose, jasmine, neroli, and tuberose are extremely expensive and are always sold in small amounts. Be very suspicious of such oils offered at a relatively low price.

♦ Established companies with a solid reputation are more likely to have reliable sources and better buying power and therefore offer quality at competitive prices.

FOUR

The Chemistry of
Essential Oils

THE ATOMIC SAGA

Atoms consist of electrons, which have a negative electrical charge, orbiting around a nucleus. The nucleus contains the protons, which have a positive electrical charge, and the neutrons, with no electric charge. Each atom has the same number of electrons and protons, to bring the total electrical charge to zero. The electrons are disposed in layers around the nucleus. Each layer can hold a set maximum number of electrons. Thus, the first layer cannot contain more than two electrons, the second layer holds a maximum of eight electrons, and so on.

Hydrogen is the most common atom in the universe and has the simplest possible structure. A single electron orbiting around one proton; it has one empty space in its single layer. Carbon, another very common atom, consists of six protons and six neutrons in the nucleus, with six orbiting electrons—two in its first layer, four in its second layer—and four empty spaces.

Oxygen has eight neutrons, eight protons, and eight electrons—two in its first layer, six in its second layer—and two empty spaces.

Atoms are impelled to fill up all their electronic layers. In fact, they compusively need to fill up this outermost layer. If they are left alone, they usually combine with themselves. The hydrogen atoms share their electrons two by two; two oxygen atoms get together and each contribute two electrons. Carbons are a little bit different. Carbon atoms arrange themselves in three-dimensional patterns, each carbon being attached to four other carbons and contributing one electron to each liaison. Billions of billions of carbon atoms can thus be connected in huge patterns.

But most atoms seem to prefer diversity. They combine with other atoms to form molecules in a kind of atomic mating process, called bonding. Atomic bonding consists of sharing the electrons in the outermost layer so as to fill up this layer. When two atoms share one electron in a molecular liaison, it is called a single bond. Atoms may also share two electrons in a double bond or even three electrons in a triple bond.

Hydrogen can form only a single bond; oxygen can form single bonds (as in water, where it is attached to two hydrogens) or double bonds (as in carbon dioxide, where two oxygens share two electrons each with a carbon). Carbon can form triple bonds, usually with itself.

By human standards, atomic behavior can be rather objectionable and creepy: to fill up their outmost layer, atoms will use any possible means. They tear molecules apart to steal others' atoms, which is called an atomic reaction. And some atomic reactions can be pretty wild. Thus when you send, for instance, some oxygen atoms into a crowd of methane molecules (each made of four hydrogens attached to one carbon), the oxygen atoms are so anxious to combine that any spark causes an explosion. The oxygens split the methane; some oxygens join with hydrogens to create plain water, while others take care of the carbons in carbon dioxide. The whole exchange is brief but rather intense. This is exactly what happens when a gas leak blows up a ten-story building.

When the universe was still young and reckless, the type of atomic massacre that I just described was really nothing compared to what was going on every day. As time went by, atoms settled down in more stable molecules (burned out, probably). The interchanges became more sophisticated, especially on our planet. Molecules got bigger and bigger, until life became possible. From general warfare,

atomic behavior evolved into a harmonious dance. Under the tight control of life forces, molecules go around, gently swapping atoms or atomic groups.

Carbon is the major performer in life's molecular dance. Its blatant promiscuity and its ability to link with itself allow it to generate chains of carbon atoms. In such chains, each carbon atom is linked to one (at each end of the chain) or two (inside the chain) carbon atoms. Carbons usually attach themselves to each other through a single bond. This leaves space for two or three extra bonds where hydrogen and oxygen (carbon's two major partners in life's waltz) or other radicals can be attached. Molecules as complex as DNA, life's inner memory chip, can thus be created.

The smaller molecules tend to be volatile—that is, they evaporate easily. The larger the molecule, the lower its ability to evaporate (i.e., the higher its boiling point). Essential oils are volatile; their molecules are rather small. Most of them have ten or fifteen carbon atoms (see discussion in next section of terpenoid molecules).

THE CHEMISTRY OF COMMON ESSENTIAL OIL CONSTITUENTS*

Almost all of the molecules found in essential oils are composed of carbon and hydrogen or of carbon, hydrogen, and oxygen. The chemistry of the constituents of essential oils is determined by two factors,

* In collaboration with Kurt Schnaubelt, Ph.D.

one artificial (the steam distillation process) and the other intrinsic to the plant (the biosynthesis of the constituent molecules).

By steam distillation, a process that is mainly physical, only volatile and water-insoluble constituents are isolated from the plant. The main types of chemical compounds isolated are terpenes, terpenoid compounds, and phenylpropane-derived compounds. There are many other constituents in plants (often valuable) that do not find their way into the essential oils. Among them are all the molecules that are soluble in water, like acids or sugars, or that are too large or too high in polarity to evaporate with steam, such as tannins, flavonoids, carotenoids, and polysaccharides. Three main categories of chemical compounds can therefore be distinguished in essential oils: (1) terpenes and terpenoid compounds; (2) sesquiterpenes and sesquiterpenoid compounds; and (3) phenylopropane derivatives. The first two share the same biosynthetic pathway.

Terpenes and Sesquiterpenes

Terpenes and sesquiterpenes are molecules made up of carbon and hydrogen (hydrocarbons). They provide the basic chemical structures through the ability of the carbon atom to form chemical bonds with other carbon atoms. Carbon atoms bonding to each other determine much of the overall shape and size of the molecule—they form the "carbon backbone" of the molecule. If the only other element present is hydrogen, the molecules are called unsubstituted and are referred to as terpenes or sesquiterpenes.

The terpenoid molecules share a common biosynthetic pathway. Their chemical structure can be looked at as if they were made up of multiples of the isoprene molecule. The isoprene structure consists of a chain of five carbon atoms. (Rationalizing the makeup of terpenoid molecules as multiples of isoprene units is a useful model, but the actual biosynthesis takes a different course.) The smallest molecules formed in this way are the monoterpenes, with ten carbon atoms. They are the main constituents of many essential oils.

Molecules with fifteen carbon atoms, sesquiterpenes, are also commonly encountered in essential oils, since they are still volatile enough to distill with steam. Molecules with twenty carbons (diterpenes) are found in essential oils to a much lesser degree. Terpenoid molecules with thirty and forty carbon atoms also occur in plants but are not found in the essential oils. Their molecular weight is too high to allow evaporation with steam. Important molecules of life like steroids and certain hormones are members of this last group. Monoterpenes have a ten-carbon structure, sesquiterpenes have fifteen carbons, and diterpenes have twenty carbons.

Functional Groups in Essential Oil Constituents

Unsubstituted hydrocarbons can be modified by a functional group; that is, one or two hydrogen atoms are replaced by the functional group in the molecule.

Within the realm of essential oils, the functional groups we have to deal with are all formed through the different ways oxygen can be attached to carbon.

Generally, molecules made up of a terpene structure and a functional group are called terpenoid (or sesquiterpenoid, from sesquiterpenes). Strictly speaking, the term terpenes (or sesquiterpenes) would refer to hydrocarbons and terpenoid to substituted terpenes. In the professional literature, the terpene (or sesquiterpene) is often used to denote the whole group of molecules with the same basic structure, including hydrocarbons and substituted molecules.

The properties of essential oil constituents are determined by their basic structure (mono-, sesqui-, and diterpene) and their functional group (Figure 3).

Ketones (Figure 3a)

Thujone, pulegone, pinocamphone, and carvone are important ketones. Oxygen can be attached to a carbon through a double bond. The resulting group is called a carboxyl group; if the oxygen is attached to a carbon located within carbonic chain, the resulting molecule is called a ketone.

Monoterpenoid ketones determine the main characteristics of a fair number of essential oils, such as hyssop and sage. Other oils with a substantial ketone content are thuja and pennyroyal (neither should ever be taken internally). The applications of these oils most relevant to aromatherapy are easing or increasing the flow of mucus and their cytophylactic effect. Both properties are utilized extensively in aromatherapy in remedies for upper respiratory complaints (mucolytic)

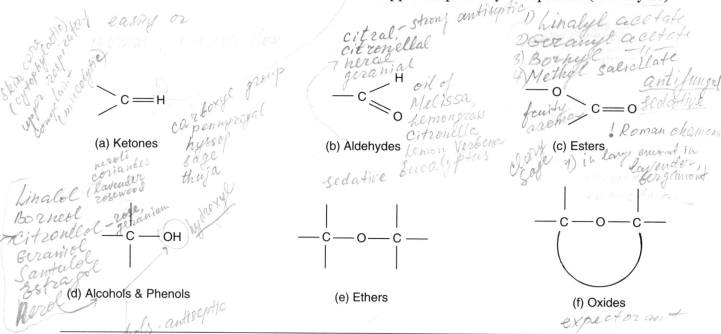

Fig. 3. Functional Groups in Essential Oil Constuents
(C, Carbon; H, Hydrogen; O, Oxygen)

and skin care preparations (cytophylactic). Many ketones are neurotoxic when taken internally. Some of them can be dangerous (pulegone in pennyroyal, thujone in mugwort, *Sage officinali,* and thuja).

Aldehydes (Figure 3b)

Citral, citronellal, neral, and geranial are important aldehydes. Like ketones, aldehydes have a carboxyl group, but unlike the ketone, their oxygen is attached to a carbon that is also linked to a hydrogen, which means that they are not located with a carbonic chain.

Monoterpenoid aldehydes are the main chemical feature of the oils of melissa (*Melissa officinalis*), lemongrass, citronella, lemon verbena (*Lippia citriodora*), and *Eucalyptus citriodora.* Studies show that aldehydes found in these oils are sedative. Citral has also been found to possess strong antiseptic properties.

Esters (Figure 3c)

Linalyl acetate, geranyl acetate, bornyl acetate, and methyl salicilate are important esters. Ester groups contain a double bond between carbon and oxygen (carboxyl group). A second oxygen molecule is bonded to the carboxyl group, rendering it an ester group. Esters are produced through the reaction of an alcohol and an acid. Esters are characteristically antifungal and sedative. They have a direct calming effect on the central nervous system and can be powerful spasmolytic agents.

Roman chamomile contains a number of esters that are not found commonly in other essential oils. The spasmolytic power apparently reaches a maximum in this oil.

Esters are generally fragrant and often have very fruity aromas. They are commonly used in compositions of fruit aromas and flavorings. Linalyl acetate, for instance, is found in large amounts in lavender and bergamot. It is the reaction product of linalol and acetic acid. Clary sage is another oil whose ester characteristics are obvious, especially if it is used in massage.

Esters are found in essential oils in probably larger numbers than the representatives of any of the other groups. Few essential oils have esters as the main constituent, but often even small amounts of characteristic esters are crucial to the finer notes in the fragrance of an essential oil.

Terpene Alcohols (Figure 3d)

Linalol, borneol, citronellol, geraniol, santalol, estragol, and nerol are important alcohols. Oxygen is most often attached to a terpene molecule through a single bond in the hydroxyl group, in which a hydrogen takes up the second oxygen bond. The hydroxyl group (–O–H) consists of a water molecule (H–O–H) separated from one of its hydrogen carbons, hence its name. The hydroxyl group has very strong reactive power.

Molecules with a hydroxyl group are called alcohols. They are typically very fluid. If an alcohol group is introduced into a terpene molecule, the resulting compound is called an alcohol or terpene alcohol. Terpene alcohols are among the most useful molecules in aromatherapy. The terpene alcohols found in common essential oils show a fair degree of diversity with respect to their properties as well as their fragrance, but also have several properties in common. Terpene alcohols are generally antiseptic, and a positive energizing effect is attributed to them. Linalol is a prominent terpene alcohol in lavender, rosewood, petitgrain, neroli, and coriander. Citronellol, which has been shown to possess antiviral qualities, is a main constituent in rose and geranium oils, and geraniol is found in palmarosa. Alpha-terpineol is characteristic in *Eucalyptus radiata* and niaouli (*Melaleuca viridiflora*). Terpineol-4 is a main constituent in tea tree and garden marjoram. Other oils also in this group are present in *Ravensare aromatica* and cajeput.

All these oils have as common qualities an antiseptic nature; a pleasant, uplifting fragrance; desirable properties; and very low toxicity. The usefulness of the terpene alcohols has been pointed out again through research that suggests that those juniper oils with a high terpineol-4 content and a corresponding low content of pinenes (terpene hydrocarbons) are the safest diuretic agents among the different types of juniper oil.

Cineol (Figure 3f)

If oxygen links two carbons and at the same time is a member of a ring structure, the compound is called an oxide. Cineol, also called eucalyptole, is almost in a class of its own. As a chemical compound it is an oxide. It imparts a strong expectorant effect to the different varieties of eucalyptus oils. It is practically ubiquitous, being a more or less desired constituent of almost every other essential oil.

Linalol oxide is an important constituent of the oil of the decumbent variety of *Hyssopus officinalis*. This oil has a low ketone content and a reduced toxicity compared with the oil of *Hyssopus officinalis*.

Phenols

Thymol, carvacrol, and eugenol are shown in Figure 4. When an alcohol hydroxyl group is attached to a benzene ring, the resulting compound is called a phenol. The phenol structure is strongly electropositive and therefore very active chemically. Phenols like thymol or carvacrol are the strongest antibacterial agents among the monoterpenoid compounds of aromatherapy.

Their strongly stimulant character is widely utilized in aromatherapy; however, these oils can be very irritating, and they should be used only in appropriately low concentrations.

Phenylpropane Derivatives

Eugenol, cinnamic aldehyde, anethol, methylchavicol, safrol, myristicin, and apiol are shown in Figure 4 (also see Table 1). The common characteristic of this class of essential oil constituents is that they are all derived from the phenylpropane structure. The elements that make up this structure are an "aromatic" phenyl ring system with a propane (three-carbon) side chain. This basic structure of nine carbon atoms is then modified by various groups attached to it. A double bond in the side chain often allows the attached groups to interact with the pi-electron system of the aromatic ring, rendering some molecules in this group pharmacologically highly active. Their biosynthetic pathway, originating

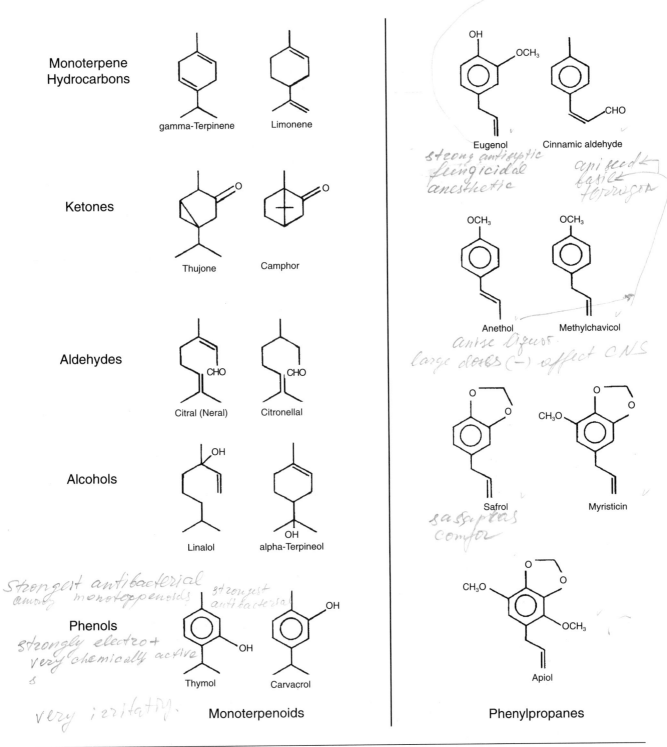

Monoterpene
Hydrocarbons

gamma-Terpinene   Limonene

Ketones

Thujone   Camphor

Aldehydes

Citral (Neral)   Citronellal

Alcohols

Linalol   alpha-Terpineol

Phenols

Thymol   Carvacrol

Monoterpenoids

Eugenol   Cinnamic aldehyde

Anethol   Methylchavicol

Safrol   Myristicin

Apiol

Phenylpropanes

Handwritten notes:
- Cinnamon / clove — strong antiseptic
- strong antiseptic / fungicidal / anesthetic (Eugenol)
- aniseed / basil / fennel (Anethol/Methylchavicol)
- anise liquor. / large doses (—) effect CNS
- sassafras / camfor (Safrol)
- Strongest antibacterial among monoterpenoids (Thymol)
- strongest antibacterial (Carvacrol)
- strongly electro+ / very chemically active / very irritating.

Fig. 4. Examples of Terpene and Phenylpropane Essential Oil Constituents

through shikimic acid, is different from those of the terpenoids.

Cinnamon and clove, like the phenolic essence, are strong antiseptic agents. They can cause severe skin reactions and must be used with caution. Eugenol, the main constituent of clove oil, in addition to being antiseptic and fungicidal, shows local anesthetic properties. It has also been reported to inhibit certain carcinogenic processes. The same effect was found for caryophyllen, another constituent of clove oil (see sesquiterpenes). Aniseed, basil, and tarragon are not as aggressive as cinnamon or clove can be, yet they all share a distinctly sweet character in their fragrance. The main constituents of basil and aniseed oils, methylchavicol and anethol, can cause negative effects if used in unreasonably high concentrations.

Others in this group include safrol (sassafras, camphor), myristicin (nutmeg), and apiol (parsley). While most of these oils can be used beneficially in aromatherapy, they share a potential for toxicity in high concentrations or with prolonged use. The potential of nutmeg to act as a hallucinogen (dosages required to induce these effect are unsafe and can cause lasting damage or death) and the effects of anethol, well known through its abuses in anise liqueurs, demonstrate the ability of phenylpropane constituents to interact with the central nervous system in a way that depends strongly on dosage and/or concentration.

Many of the properties of terpenoid essential oil constituents (ketones, aldehydes, terpene alcohols, esters, cineol, and phenols) are listed in Table 2.

Table 1
Properties of Phenylpropane-Derived Essential Oil Constituents

Phenylpropane derivative	Property	Source
Eugenol	Antiseptic	Clove
Cinnamic aldehyde	Stimulant, skin irritant	Cinnamon
Anethol	Increase secretion	Aniseed
Methylchavicol	Expectorant Spasmolytic	Basil, tarragon Parsley, nutmeg, sassafras
Safrol, myristicin, apiol	Diuretic, spasmolytic, abortive (apiol), central nervous system stimulant, hallucinogenic (myristicin)	

Table 2
Properties of Terpenoid Essential Oil Constituents

Terpenoid	Property	Source
Ketones	Promote tissue formation, mucolytic, potentially neurotoxic	Sage, thuja, wormwood (thujone), hyssop (pinocamphone)
Aldehydes	Anti-inflammative, sedative, antiviral	Melissa, lemongrass (citrals), citronella, *Eucalyptus citriodora* (citronella)
Terpene alcohols	Bactericidal, toning, diuretic, antiviral	Lavender, coriander, petitgrain, rosewood (linalol), *Eucalyptus radiata*, niaouli (alpha-terpineol), tea tree, marjoram, juniper (terpineol-4)
Esters	Spasmolytic, sedative, can be antifungal	Roman chamomile (angelica acid esters), lavender, clary sage, bergamot (linalyl acetate)
Cineol	Expectorant	Eucalyptus and many other oils
Phenols	Bactericidal, immunostimulant, stimulant, skin irritant, potentially toxic to liver	Thyme (thymol), oregano, savory (carvacrol)

Terpene Hydrocarbons

Limonene (90 percent or more of most citrus oils), pinene, camphene, and myrcene are shown in Figure 4. With regard to their properties, terpene hydrocarbons are often thought to be rather insignificant constituents of essential oils. There has been discussion of whether terpenes are skin or mucous membrane irritants. Studies of various pine oils show that antiseptic principles are formed when these oils are subjected to natural or induced aging or oxidation. A study of the effects of terpenes against Herpes simplex and other viruses should renew the respect for terpenes in aromatherapy. Limonene, the main constituent of many citrus oils; alpha-sabinene; and gamma-terpinene have

Table 3
General Effects of Terpenoid Compounds*

Activity	Monoterpenes	Sesquiterpenes	Diterpenes
Anesthetic	+		
Analeptic	+	+	
Analgesic		+	
Anthelmintic	+	+	
Antiarrythmic		+	
Antibiotic	+	+	+
(antibacterial, antifungal, antiseptic, antiviral)			
Antiepileptic		+	
Antihistaminic	+		
Anti-inflammatory, antiphlogistic	+	+	
Antirheumatic	+		
Antitumor	+	+	+
(antiblastic, anticarcinogenic, cytotoxic)			
Chloeretic, choloagogue		+	
Diuretic	+		
Expectorant	+		+
Hypotensive	+	+	+
Insecticidal	+		+
Irritant	+	+	
Juvenile hormone		+	
Pheromone	+	+	
Phytohormone		+	+
(growth regulating)			
Purgative	+		+
Sedative	+	+	
Spasmolytic	+	+	
Toxic		+	+
Vitamin			+

*The biological, pharmacological, and therapeutical activity of normal monoterpenes (and also of many sesquiterpenes) is closely connected to that of the essential oils. An overview of the most important biological properties of mono-, sesqui-, and diterpenes is given here.

all been found to possess antiviral properties. Essential oils with high proportions of monoterpene hydrocarbons include:

Lemon, orange, bergamot (limonene)
Black pepper (pinenes, camphenes, etc.)
Pine oils (pinenes)
Turpentine (pinenes, limonene)
Nutmeg (pinenes)
Mastick (pinenes)
Angelica (pinenes)

Table 3 illustrates the activities of monoterpenes, as well as sesquiterpenes and diterpenes.

Sesquiterpenes

Chamazulen, bisabolol, santalol, zingiberol, carotol, caryophyllen, and farnesol are among the important sesquiterpenes. Table 4 lists some sources of sesquiterpenes.

As we look at sesquiterpene constituents of essential oils, the influence of a functional group becomes less dominating. The increased size of the overall structure brings about increased complexity. The interaction between carbon backbone and functional group becomes more subtle and intricate. The individuality of the molecule becomes a greater factor in the makeup of the pharmacological effect of the molecule.

Table 4
Sources of Sesquiterpenes in Essential Oils

Sesquiterpene	Property	Source
		From roots
Zingiberol		Ginger
Vetiveron, vetiverol	Stomachic, carminative	Vetiver
Complex composition (almost 100% sesquiterpenes)		Spikenard
Valeranon (valepotriates C 101)	Sedative, spasmolytic	Valerian
		From woods, seeds, or leaves
Alpha-Santalol		Sandalwood
Patchouli alcohol		Patchouli
Carotol		Carrot seed
Nerolidol (dependent on type)	Disinfectant, antiseptic	Niaouli
		From the plant family asteraceae
Chamazulene, bisabolol	Antiphlogistic *anti inflamatory*	German chamomile
Chamazulene (dependent on chemotype)		Yarrow
Chamazulene (dependent on chemotype)		Tansy

More than two thousand sesquiterpenes have been isolated from plants to date, and their structures vary widely. Most of these sesquiterpenes can be attributed to thirty main structural types. A summary of their biological activity is shown in Table 5. Essential oils with a high proportion of sesquiterpene constituents are mostly distilled from roots and woods or from plants of the Asterceae family.

Sesquiterpenes have been the object of much interest and research into their properties. The bulk of that research has been performed on sesquiterpenes isolated from plants of the Asterceae family that are not common essential oil plants. The situation for the aromatherapist is somewhat unsatisfactory, since there are good reasons to speculate on the potential properties of sesquiterpenes in essential oils, but only limited availability of substantiating research data. There are some notable exceptions. In the effort to provide a scientific basis for the many uses of German chamomile (*Chamomilla matricaria*), the antiphlogistic properties of chamazulene and alpha-bisabolol were firmly established.

Farnesol is a sesquiterpene whose superior properties as a bacteriostatic and dermatophilic agent are well documented. Because of its ability to inhibit, rather than kill, the growth of bacteria, it is an ideal deodorizing agent, since it inhibits the development of odor-causing micro-organisms without eliminating the bacteria that are present on healthy skin.

Finally, caryophyllen, which is found in many essential oils, most notably in clove oil, has received renewed attention. It combines sedative and antiviral effects with an ability to inhibit some carcinogenic processes.

Sandalwood illustrates the lack of solid research data on sesquiterpenes that are found in essential oils. On one hand there is ample anecdotal evidence for its usefulness in urinary tract infections, and even pharmacological textbooks list it as a potential urine disinfectant. On the

Table 5
Sesquiterpenes from Essential Oils with Known Pharmacological Properties

Sesquiterpene	*Property*	*Source*
Chamazulene	Antiphlogistic, anti-inflammatory	German chamomile, yarrow, tansy
Caryophyllen	Sedative, antiviral potentially anticarcinogenic	Clove (10%); occurs in many essential oils in low concentrations
Farnesol	Bacteriostatic	Rose, chamomile, and many other flower oils

other hand, an antibacterial effect of sandalwood oil constituents has not been confirmed. It is of course tempting to speculate that searching for an outright bactericidal effect of santalol may be the wrong experiment in light of the fact that sesquiterpenes can be effective immune stimulants. The effect of the oil could be caused not through direct bactericidal action but rather through stimulation of the body's defense mechanisms. A summary of essential oils and their major chemical components is given in Table 6.

Table 6
Essential Oils and Their Major Chemical Components

Plant	*Number of carbons*	*Components*
Angelica	10	Musk ketone
Aniseed	9	Phenylpropane (*trans*-anethole)
Basil	9	Phenylpropane (methylchavicol)
Bay		Phenylpropanes: myrcene, eugenol, charvical
Bergamot	10	Terpenes and esters: limonene, linalyl acetate
Birch		Esters: methyl salicilate
Cajeput	10	Terpene alcohols: alpha-terpineol
Caraway	10	Ketones: limonen, carvone
Cardamom	10	Terpenes: cineol
Carrot seed	15	Sesquiterpene alcohol: carotol
Cedarwood		Ketone: atlantone-7
Chamomile, blue		Sesquiterpenoids: chamazulene
Chamomile, German	15	Sesquiterpenoids: bisabolol, chamazulene
Chamomile, mixta		Alcohol: ormenol
Chamomile, Roman		Esters
Champaca, *Michelia alba*		Terpene alcohol
Cinnamon bark	9	Phenylpropane: cinnamic aldehyde
Cinnamon leaf	9	Phenylpropane: eugenol
Cistus		Terpenes, sesquiterpenes, diterpenes
Citronella	10	Aldehydes: citronellal
Clary sage		Esters: linalyl acetate, sesquiterpene alcohol
Clove buds	9	Phenylpropane-phenol, eugenol
Coriander seeds		Terpene alcohols: linalol
Cumin seeds		Aldehyde: cuminaldehyde
Cypress	10	Terpenes: terpenyl acetate
Elemi	10	Terpenes: limonene, elemol
Eucalyptus australiana		Cineol
Eucalyptus citriodora		Aldehydes: citronellal
Eucalyptus globulus	10	Cineole, *t*-alcohol
Everlasting		Esters: neryl esters

Table 6 (continued)

Plant	Number of carbons	Components
Fennel		Phenylpropane: *trans*-anethole
Fir	10	Terpenes
Frankincense	10	Terpenes: phellandrene, camphene, olibanol
Geranium	10	Alcohols: citronellol, geraniol
Ginger root	15	Sesquiterpenoids: zingiberone
Grapefruit	10	Terpenes: limonene
Hyssop	10	Ketone: pinocarvone
Jasmine		Benzyl acetate, jasmine
Juniper	10	Terpenes, terpene alcohol
Laurel	10	Cineole
Lavender	10	Esters, terpene alcohols: linalyl acetate
Lavandin	10	Esters, terpene alcohols: linalol, camphor, linalyl acetate
Lemon	10	Terpenes, aldehyde: limonene, citral
Lemongrass	10	Aldehyde: citral
Lime	10	Terpenes, aldehyde: limonen, citral
Litsea cubeba	10	Aldehyde: citrals
Lovage root		Lactones
Marjoram	10	Terpene alcohols: terpine-4-ol
Marjoram, wild Spanish	10	Phenol
Melissa	10	Aldehyde, citrals
Mugwort	10	Ketone: thujone
Myrrh	10	Terpenes
Myrtle	10	Terpenes, terpene alcohols
Neroli	10	Terpene alcohols, esters: linalol, geraniol, nerol
Niaouli	10	Terpenes, terpene alcohols
Nutmeg	9	Terpenes, alcohols: linalol, borneol, myristicin
Orange	10	Terpenes
Oregano	10	Phenol: carvacrol
Palmarosa	10	Terpene alcohols: geraniol
Patchouli	15	Sesquiterpenoids: patchoulol
Pennyroyal	10	Ketone: pulegone, methone
Pepper	10	Terpenes: piperine
Peppermint	10	Terpene alcohols: menthol, carvone, linalol
Petitgrain biguarade	10	Terpenes, esters: linalyl acetate
Pine	10	Terpenes
Rose	10	Alcohols: citronellol, geraniol, nerol
Rosemary	10	Terpenes, terpene alcohols: cineol
Rosewood	10	Terpene alcohols: linalol
Sage lavandulifolia	10	Cineole, camphor, esters
Sandalwood, Mysore	15	Sesquiterpenoids: santalol
Savory	10	Phenol: carvacrol
Spearmint	10	Terpene alcohols: carvone

Table 6 (continued)

Plant	Number of carbons	Components
Spike	10	Terpene alcohols: linalol, camphor
Spikenard		Sesquiterpene alcohol
Spruce	10	Terpenes
Tangerine	10	Terpenes
Tarragon	9	Phenylpropane: methylchavicol
Tea tree	10	Terpenes, terpene alcohols: terpinen-4-ol
Therebentine	10	Terpenes: p-menthadienes
Thyme, citriodora		Aldehyde: citral
Thyme, lemon		Alcohol: linalol
Thyme, red		Phenol: thymol
Verbena, lemon	10	Aldehyde: citrals
Vetiver	15	Sesquiterpenoids: vetiveron, vetiverol
Ylang-ylang		Alcohols: geraniol, linalol, ylangol

FIVE

Principles of Aromatherapy:
How Essential Oils Work

Aromatherapy is rather different from other healing modalities in that it acts on various levels, each in synergy with the other levels. Aromatherapy treats symptoms by addressing the specific physical, energetic, and psychological background of the individual client.

BIOPHYSICAL ACTION OF ESSENTIAL OILS

Essential oils have measurable biophysical actions when inhaled, ingested, or applied to the body. There are some general properties that we find to a greater or a lesser degree in all essential oils, due to the fact that essential oils are made primarily of terpenoid compounds. However, each individual essential oil has specific properties due to its specific chemical composition.

Healers and pharmacists have long made use of essential oils' biophysical actions. Essential oils have been used in pharmaceutical preparations since the beginning of pharmacy in Egypt more than six thousand years ago and are still used in Europe, Asia, and the United States today. In France, cough preparations, digestive aids, muscle liniments, and wound preparations found in virtually every pharmacy contain essential oils as active ingredients. In the United States, "Vick's Vapo-Rub" includes peppermint, eucalyptus, and several other essential oils as active ingredients. In Asia, Tiger Balm is made primarily of essential oils.

Medicinal Properties Found in Most Essential Oils

Antiseptic Property
A property universally found in essential oils is the antiseptic property. All essential oils are antiseptic to some degree. The most antiseptic are the oils with a high phenolic content. Phenolic compounds

found in essential oils are thymol, carvacrol, and eugenol. These compounds are found in especially large quantities in red thyme, savory, oregano, clove, and cinnamon. Such oils are extremely powerful antiseptics, but should be used with caution, since they can be irritating, especially when applied to the skin. Phenol-rich essential oils should be used only under medical supervision.

In addition to the very aggressive phenolic oils, aromatherapy provides us with a wide choice of milder but very effective essential oils for antiseptic use. These include all the oils rich in alcohols, such as geranium, all the various lavenders, palmarosa, tea tree, marjoram, and ylang-ylang. These oils are much milder than the phenol-rich oils and are very safe to use. They are useful for home remedies and first-aid kits, and they work well on minor wounds, as prevention from infectious diseases, or for skin care.

Oils rich in terpenes include pine and most of the coniferae (fir, spruce, cedarwood, juniper) and the citruses (lemon, lime, orange, grapefruit, tangerine). These oils are slightly more aggressive than the alcoholic oils, but are still very safe to use. They are especially efficient when used in a diffuser.

Expectorant

In addition to their overall antiseptic properties, most essential oils are expectorants to some degree, which means that they stimulate the fluidification and expulsion of mucus from the lungs. As we know, the lungs produce mucus to filter the air that we breathe. Mucus traps the dust and pollutants that we breathe all day long. It is very important that we expel mucus properly, especially when we live in polluted cities. Essential oils are helpful for this purpose.

The most effective expectorant oils are those that are rich in a chemical called cineol and include most of the myrtaceae (eucalyptus, myrtle, niaouli, cajeput) and the coniferae (pine, spruce, fir, cedarwood). Eucalyptus globulus is one of the most powerful expectorants.

Cytophilactic

Most essential oils are cytophilactic, which means that they stimulate cellular activity and cellular regeneration. The most cytophilactic oils are geranium, lavender, rosemary, sandalwood, and, generally, all the oils rich in alcohol.

Rubefacient

Essential oils are rubefacient, which means that they activate capillary circulation. This is especially true of oils rich in phenols (thyme, oregano, savory, clove) and, to a lesser degree, oils rich in oxides (eucalyptus, niaouli, cajeput, rosemary) and terpenes (pine, fir, juniper).

Major Medicinal Properties of Individual Essential Oils

Each essential oil also has specific properties, depending on its chemical composition. The major medicinal properties found in some essential oils are listed in Table 7.

Table 7
Medicinal Properties of Individual Essential Oils

Property	Essential oils
Sedative/calming	Neroli, spikenard, lavender, chamomile, marjoram, ylang-ylang
Energizing/stimulant	Peppermint, ginger, nutmeg, pepper, rosemary, lemon, eucalyptus, pine
Antispasmodic (cramps, colics, PMS, cough)	Cypress, Roman chamomile, tarragon, lavender
Anti-inflammatory	Blue and Roman chamomile, helycrisum
Emmenagogue (regulates female hormonal system)	German chamomile, clary sage, fennel, mugwort, lavender
Aphrodisiac	Jasmine, champaca flowers, ylang-ylang, clary sage, sandalwood, patchouli, cistus, pepper
Analgesic/pain killer	Clove, birch, red thyme, rosemary

ACTION OF ESSENTIAL OILS ON THE SKIN

Essential oils are extremely beneficial for the skin. In fact, the use of essential oils in skin care can be traced back to the Egyptians, the inventors of cosmetology. The Egyptians had extremely elaborate skin care regimens, which could take hours to complete. Their skin care preparations made extensive use of aromatic substances.

The skin is a barrier between our bodies and the outside world. Thus, the skin absorbs and filters elements from the air and absorbs a small amount of air (the skin breathes). It also absorbs moisture and other elements applied to the skin. The skin must filter germs and unwanted substances such as pollutants. This double function of the skin is extremely important. At the same time, our bodies expel moisture to help control body temperature. The skin expels sebum, a waxy substance that our bodies use as a protectant; it also expels various waste materials through the sebaceous glands.

Essential oils help the skin to perform its role as a barrier. This is a very important property for skin care. In addition, some of the basic properties of essential oils make them extremely useful for skin care.

ACTION OF ESSENTIAL OILS ON THE ENERGY LEVEL

Essential oils are considered the life force, the energy, of the plant. They are used with great efficiency in energy work such as acupressure, Shiatsu, and chakra work. Specific essential oils can be associated with each meridian and chakra. See Tables 8, 9, and 10.

Table 8
Action of Essential Oils on the Skin

Property	Essential oils	Special applications
Antiseptic	Tea tree, eucalyptus, niaouli, lavender, geranium	Cleansing, protecting and treating acne-prone skin*
Cytophilactic/ cellular stimulant	Myrrh, frankincense, rose, sandalwood, geranium, rosemary, lavender	Treatment and healing of minor skin lesions and blemishes, mature skin
Rubefacient	Juniper, grapefruit, rosemary, red thyme (in very small doses)	Toxin elimination, lymphatic drainage, treatment of sluggish conditions
Astringent	Geranium, lemongrass, lemon	Skin toner, treatment of oily skin
Regulator	Sage	Sebaceous secretions, oily skin
Protectant	Palmarosa, sandalwood, myrrh	Protect skin, help it retain moisture
Soother	Chamomile, neroli, rosewood, rose, ylang-ylang	Sensitive skin Couperose, broken capillaries

Caution: Do not use oregano or clove on skin; use red thyme only in very low concentration on skin.

Table 9
Essential Oils and Meridians (Refer to a Meridian Chart)

Meridian	Essential oils
Lungs	Oils of the myrtaceae family (Eucalyptus globulus, Australiana and smithii, myrtle, niaouli, cajeput), coniferae family (fir, pine, spruce, cedarwood, cypress), hyssop, lavender
Liver	Sage, rosemary, lemon, peppermint, chamomile
Stomach	Oils of the umbelliferae family (aniseed, angelica, fennel, caraway, coriander, tarragon), ginger, orange, peppermint, chamomile
Intestine	Savory, cinnamon (bark and leaf), ginger, angelica, tarragon, fennel, caraway, coriander, cardamom

Table 10
Essential Oils and Chakras (Refer to a Chakra Chart)

Chakra	Essential oils
Root	Vetiver, spikenard, angelica, ginger, cedarwood, spruce
Sex	Jasmine, champaca flowers, ylang-ylang, pepper, clary sage, patchouli, sandalwood
Solar plexus	Rosemary, ginger, nutmeg, sage, pepper, thyme
Heart	Neroli, rose, marjoram, melissa
Throat	Geranium, eucalyptus
Third eye	Mugwort, sandalwood, cedarwood, vetiver
Crown	Cistus, rose, jasmine, sandalwood, spikenard

ACTION OF ESSENTIAL OILS ON THE EMOTIONAL LEVEL

Essential oils are first and foremost fragrances, and as such they have deep effects on the emotional plane. Table 11 describes what essential oils to use to influence specific moods.

ACTION OF ESSENTIAL OILS ON THE SPIRITUAL PLANE

Aromatic substances have been used for ritualistic purposes since the origins of human culture. It was, in fact, one of their first uses. Traditional cultures viewed fragrances as a link between the human realm and the gods. Fragrances in most ancient cultures were considered a gift from the gods. The shaman or priest used them to carry their offerings to the kingdom of the gods. Even to this day, all major religions, whether Shintoism, Buddhism, Hinduism, Islam, or Christianity, use incenses and scented oils in their rituals and ceremonies.

Essential oils, especially the oils from woods and gums, have a very centering and opening effect on the psyche. They help create a sense of connectedness, community, and elevation, and they inspire the sacred in each of us. The major oils for ritualistic purposes are sandalwood, cistus, myrrh, frankincense, benzoin, vetiver, spikenard, and rose.

When Mary Magdalene wanted to express her devotion to the Christ, she washed his feet with the famous nard oil (now known as spikenard), one of the most expensive oils of antiquity, brought by caravans from the Himalayas to Palestine. She incidentally spent a fortune on Christ's feet, provoking the hanger of Judas, the bookkeeper of the group.

This episode from the Bible inspired a blend that I created more than ten years ago, when a French religious group asked me to create a Good Friday blend to re-

Table 11
Action of Essential Oils on the Emotional Level

Mood	Essential oils
Gratifying/indulging/ warming/loving	Jasmine, ylang-ylang, rose, neroli, sandalwood, absolutes of tuberose, mimosa, narcissus, champaca flowers
Vitality/stimulating	Rosemary, juniper, peppermint, basil, coniferae, myrtaceae
Balancing/calming/ soothing	Lavender, marjoram, chamomile, neroli, ylang-ylang, tangerine, melissa, spikenard
Mental concentration, centering/deepening	Bursearaceae (myrrh, frankincense, elemi), sandalwood, cistus, spruce, coniferae
Clarifying/sharpening (for confusion)	Petitgrain, peppermint, basil, rosemary, myrtaceae
Memory stimulation	Juniper, basil, rosemary
Emotional shock, grief	Rose, neroli, marjoram, clary sage, chamomile
Stress	Chamomile, neroli, marjoram, lavender, ylang-ylang
Sadness	Benzoin, jasmine, rose, clary sage
Dream work	Mugwort, clary sage, cistus
Psychic work	Cistus, sandalwood, spikenard, rose
To build confidence, self-esteem	Alternate between gratifying in evening and vitality in morning

enact the foot washing. I later added this blend to my line under the name *Sacred*. It combines the major ritualistic oils of all major spiritual traditions.

CONCLUSION

The various levels of action of essential oils are not exclusive from one another. On the contrary, whatever the application, we always encounter the various effects to one degree or another. When doing skin care or body care treatments in particular, there will be not only physical effects and effects on the skin, but also effects on the energy level and on the emotional level. Each level of action works in synergy with the others to enhance the overall effect.

The capacity to affect people on so many different levels—physical/medicinal, skin, energy, emotional/psychological—is really what makes aromatherapy so special. No other healing art has such versatility and broadness of action.

This capacity is also what makes aromatherapy such a creative art. The possibilities are endless: one can go as far as he or she wishes. Aromatherapy offers unique opportunities to fine tune and personalize treatments to an extreme degree. The trained technician can design treatments that take into account the client's biophysical background, skin type, energy level, and emotional and psychological state. Mastering aromatherapy is a challenging but uniquely rewarding venture.

SIX

The Use of Essential Oils for Health, Beauty, and Well-Being

Essential oils are pleasant and easy to use. They can be used in many different ways; however, particular methods are more suited to particular applications. For instance, the diffuser is the best way to treat lung conditions, while massage is the best application for muscle pain or rheumatism. The various methods of application of essential oils can be used in conjunction. Massage, bath, and diffuser, for instance, work wonders when used in combination.

The major methods of using essential oils are:

♦ *Internally (by ingestion):* Essential oils should be taken only internally under direct supervision of a physician.
♦ *Through inhalation.*
♦ *Through the skin* (massage, bath, friction, application).
♦ *Skin care and cosmetic use* (facial, compresses, masks, lotions, creams).
♦ *Hair care.*

Whether taken internally or externally, essential oils diffuse through the skin and membranes and penetrate deeply into the tissues and the circulatory system. Therefore, external application is a very efficient way to treat specific organs. As a rule, ingestion is indicated only for infectious diseases and to act on the digestive system (throat, stomach, liver, etc.). A massage of the corresponding zone is very helpful in such cases. In any case, essential oils should be taken internally only under medical supervision.

INTERNAL USE

Some adepts of aromatherapy tend to glamorize internal use. They wrongly feel that they have been initiated or have graduated to some higher level of aromatherapy when they start using essential oils internally. That attitude is reinforced by unscrupulous marketers who will market their oils as pharmaceutical grade fit for internal use, intended for the rarefied few who have been initiated to the internal art. These marketers usually charge a very stiff premium for their products.

In fact, internal use of essential oils is not safe and is not even very efficient unless they are taken in capsules or time-release form. When taken through the mouth in drops, the essential oils are mostly absorbed by the tissues in the mouth. Whatever reaches the stomach can provoke heartburn and is very hard on the liver. In fact, regular internal use of essential oils can severely damage the liver. Most of the essential oil will be destroyed in the digestive track and will never make it to the bloodstream. In the end, internal use is usually a harmful and inefficient method of application. The few reported accidents and all of the handful of fatalities from use of essential oils involved internal use.

It is true that in some cases internal use can be very efficient: two drops of peppermint oil on the tongue will quickly clear upset stomach, nausea, or motion sickness; two to three drops of rosemary on a piece of brown sugar will get rid of hangover after a wild party. Roman chamomile clears sluggish digestion or minor food poisoning. Fennel will promote lactation in nursing mothers. Likewise, cinnamon or savory in capsules are great for intestinal infections. But in most cases, internal use of essential oils strictly concerns medical practice and is generally not advised without medical supervision.

Essential oils can be taken undiluted on a small piece of sugar or mixed with honey. In this case, it is very important to carefully respect the doses. Any oil can be dangerous at high doses; the most toxic are, in decreasing order: rue, pennyroyal, thuja, lavender stoechas, mugwort, nutmeg, sage officinalis, hyssop, anise, and fennel. These oils should *never* be taken internally in any circumstances. As a rule, when other essential oils are taken internally, the maximum dose should be five drops three times a day.

For a more flexible and convenient internal use, you can dilute essential oils in ethyl alcohol (or sweet almond oil for children and people intolerant to alcohol). Mix ¼ ounce essential oils (either a single oil or a blend) in 4 ounces of 90 percent ethyl alcohol (do not use rubbing alcohol). This will give you a 5 to 6 percent preparation (for preparations in metric, use 5 to 6 milliliters of essential oil in 100 milliliters of alcohol or sweet almond oil). The average dose would be fifteen drops, three times a day, in a glass of warm water or herb tea, between meals. The maximum dose is fifty drops a day.

Aromatic honey

Mix ¼ ounce of your blend of essential oils in 16 ounces of honey for a 2 percent preparation (2 milliliters of essential oil or blend of oils in 100 milliliters of honey).

Stir thoroughly.

Dose: ½ teaspoon three times a day. (You can make a more concentrated preparation for use in capsules.)

Contraindications: Do not prescribe essential oils to be used internally by children, pregnant women, and people subject to heartburn or ulcers.

Never use the oils rich in ketone internally (thuja, pennyroyal, mugwort, hyssop, sage officinalis, lavender stoechas). Ketones, when ingested, can provoke seizure or coma and are fatal at rather low dosages.

APPLICATION OF ESSENTIAL OILS THROUGH THE OLFACTORY AND RESPIRATORY SYSTEMS

The use of aromatic fumigations is probably as old as humanity. Priests, sorcerers, and healers of all traditions used them extensively in their ceremonies and various rituals. Ancient Egyptians burned perfumes in the streets and inside the temples. More than two thousand years ago, Hippocrates, the father of western medicine, successfully struggled against the epidemic of plague in Athens, using aromatic fumigations throughout the city. In the Middle Ages, people burned pine or other fragrant woods in the streets in time of epidemic to cast out devils. Perfumers were known to resist disease.

The application of essential oils through the olfactory and respiratory systems is the easiest, most pleasant, and, in most cases, most effective way to apply them. This method requires minimal patient action: all the patient has to do is turn on a proper diffusing device, which disperses essential oils into the air, and breathe! This application method is the best and easiest way to introduce a newcomer to the world of aromatherapy.

Various devices have been designed to disperse essential oils into the air. Essential oils can be diffused in a mist with an atomizing diffuser, vaporized through heat in a candle diffuser or scented candle, or dispersed using a room spray.

Cold Diffusion

The Atomizing Diffuser

The atomizing diffuser is the most effective way to disperse essential oils into the air. It is recommended for all diseases related to the lungs, the heart, the brain, and the blood. The atomizing diffuser projects drops of essential oils into a nebulizer, using air as a propellant. The nebulizer acts as an expansion chamber, where the drops of oil are broken into a very thin mist. This mist, consisting of tiny, ionized droplets of essential oils, remains suspended for several hours, revitalizing the air with the antiseptic and deodorant properties of the essential oils. The oxidation of the essential oils provokes the formation of low doses of natural ozone that decomposes in ionic nascent oxygen. This process, occurring naturally in forests, has an invigorating and purifying effect. The atomizing diffuser is particularly effective since it diffuses the oils without altering or heating them. Since air is the propellant, there is no chemical pollution.

Through the atomizing diffuser, we experience all the various levels of action of essential oils at their maximum efficiency. It can be used for almost all prescriptions of aromatherapy. It is the subtlest, easiest, and most pleasant way to apply essential oils. It can be installed in any public or private place where air treatment is needed:

saunas, hot tubs, hospitals, consulting rooms, waiting rooms, gymnastic centers, schools, and, of course, at home, in the living room, bedroom, kitchen, or bath.

A lot of clinical research on the use of this apparatus over the last ten years demonstrates the biophysical action of essential oils applied through diffusion. In addition to the antiseptic action, already widely documented, there is a very strong action on the lungs and the respiratory system in general (asthma, bronchitis, cold, sinusitis, sore throats, etc.). The effect on the circulatory system, the heart, and the nervous system is also very pronounced.

The lungs are one of the main energy centers. Proper breathing allows for a better energy level. The absorption of essential oils through the respiratory system is one of the best ways to activate them on the energy level. There is an obvious connection between the psychic centers and the lungs. Most spiritual practices emphasize the importance of breathing. Breathing essential oils diffused through an atomizing diffuser can thus be seen as the best way to experience the subtle effects of essential oils on the emotional level, the spirit, and the soul.

Sprays

Essential oils can be dispersed into the air through a room spray. This method has the advantage of being extremely easy and portable. It can be used in many places where a diffuser is not practical (bathroom, car, garbage can, etc.). However, it creates fairly large droplets, which limit its efficiency, and, of course, it only diffuses for a fraction of a second.

Heat Diffusion

Essential oils can also be dispersed into the air through a heat source, in which case they are vaporized. This method is not as efficient as cold diffusion, which creates a mist, especially for therapeutic purposes.

Candle Diffusers

In the candle diffuser, a small candle (votive or tea light) is placed underneath a well which holds the oils. The heat vaporizes and disperses the oils.

Aromatic Candles

Aromatic candles contain 5 to 8 percent essential oils in their wax. When the wax melts, the essential oil is released. This is the most inefficient way to diffuse essential oils, because a large percentage of the oils are burned by the flame.

Dosage

The use of essential oil in a diffuser is generally very safe provided you use your common sense. For an average size room, the recommended use is fifteen to thirty minutes, two or three times a day. Permanent use can be appropriate in an open space, such as a store, or in large spaces, such as a large office, a spa, or a large house with open floor plan.

Some Oils to Use in Diffusion

The sense of smell is very subjective; you might particularly like some fragrances and dislike some others, depending on so many factors that it is impossible to tell which one will be your favorite. In addition, your appreciation will depend on your mood, the time of the day, the season, etc.

Calmer (evening): Lavender, marjoram, chamomile, tangerine
Stimulant (morning): Sage, rosemary, pine, mints
Aphrodisiac: Ylang-ylang, jasmine, champaca flowers, sandalwood, patchouli, ginger, peppermint, pepper, savory
Lungs: Eucalyptus, lavender, pine, cajeput, copaiba, hyssop
Nervousness: Mugwort, petitgrain, marjoram, neroli
Hypertension: Ylang-ylang, lavender, lemon, marjoram
Hypotension: Hyssop, sage, thyme, rosemary
Antidepressants: Frankincense, myrrh, cedarwood
Purifier: Lavandin, lemongrass, lemon, pine, chamomile, geranium, oregano
Revivifier: Pine, fir, black spruce
Brain strengthener and memory fortifier: Basil, juniper, rosemary
Insomnia: Neroli, spikenard, marjoram, chamomile

See Appendices I and II for more specific indications.

Caution

Use the diffuser with extreme caution around people subject to allergies, emphysema, or asthma, and around newborn babies. In such cases, use the diffuser for only a few minutes at a time. If any adverse reaction occurs, discontinue immediately. Do not use oils rich in ketones in the diffuser (thuja, pennyroyal, mugwort, hyssop, sage officinalis, lavender stoechas).

BODY CARE USES OF ESSENTIAL OILS

Massage

Essential oils are particularly beneficial in massage, a slow, diffuse, gentle, and pleasant way to apply them. They are completely absorbed by the skin in 60 to 120 minutes and penetrate deeply into the tissues. Their prolonged action amplifies the effects of the massage itself. Hand healing and massage are probably the most ancient healing arts, and oils, usually scented, have been part of the treatment since its beginning.

Massage goes much further than a mere tissue manipulation. It is a direct and simple form of communication between the massage therapist and patient, where the hands are extremely sensitive receptors. During the course of the massage, the hands will discover the internal geography of the body, unraveling tensions, sores, hidden pains, sensitive points, congested areas, and swollen parts, and they will tell a lot about the patient. This is why, to give the full benefit of a massage, the massage therapist must be in an open, understanding, and compassionate state of mind.

In massage, the hands are channels of healing energy; they heal at the physical, emotional, and psychic level. Therefore, aromatherapy massage is an excellent therapeutic combination as essential oils and massage have mutually enhancing effects. The massage itself will help the oils penetrate into the tissues and direct them where they are most needed, while the essential oils will treat locally or via the energy channels (nerves and meridians). You can use massage oils after the bath to moisturize and soften the skin. You can, of course, use different oils for different parts of the body, especially if you want to act on different organs.

How to Prepare a Massage Oil

Always use ultrafiltered cold-pressed or expeller oils as a base for your massage oil. If you use cold-pressed oils, it is important that the oils that you use have been ultrafiltered. Regular cold-pressed oils contain a certain amount of organic residues that will manifest as cloudiness or deposits at the bottom of the bottle. Such residues add to the richness and flavor of the oil for cooking but are undesirable for massage as they may cause pore clogging.

Sweet almond oil is the most commonly used, but it becomes rancid very easily. Grapeseed and canola oils are fine oils with a good shelf life, which easily absorb while providing a good slip, and are widely used by massage therapists and beauticians. Hazelnut oil is very rich and nourishing, although rather expensive. Peanut oil and coconut or palm oil are too heavy and may cause skin break-out. A small amount of vitamin E oil will bring some vitamins to your skin and act as a natural antioxidant.

I recommend the following oils for a massage oil base (4-ounce preparation):

Canola oil: 2 ounces
Grapeseed oil: 1.5 ounces
Wheatgerm oil: 0.5 ounces

The essential oil concentration for a massage oil depends on the type of massage and the application; see Tables 12 and 13.

Note that partial massage is massage of only one part of the body (such as shoulder massage or massage of the hips) or massage of a particular organ (stomach, liver, lungs, etc.). Topical uses are applications on a very small area such as pressure points, chakras, energy points, or meridians. Acute conditions requiring this type of application will be conditions such as rheumatism, arthritis, or tense, painful muscles.

Caution

♦ Do not use deep tissue massage on varicose or spiderweb veins. Only use gentle, light massage.

♦ Do not use oils rich in ketones, especially on pregnant women (thuja, pennyroyal, mugwort, sage officinalis, lavender stoechas).

♦ Use only very low concentrations of phenolic oils (cinnamon bark and leaf, clove, oregano, savory, red thyme).

♦ In general, it is recommended that you decrease the essential oil concentration when working on pregnant women.

♦ Always use low concentrations on young children (cut dosages in half).

♦ Do not use essential oils in massage on people undergoing chemotherapy without proper medical supervision.

Table 12
Dosage for Massage Oil

Type of massage	Recommended dose			Maximum dose		
	%	*Drops/100 ml*	*ml/100 ml*	*%*	*Drops/100 ml*	*ml/100 ml*
Full-body massage	1.5	50	1.5	4	120	4
Partial massage	3	100	3	6	200	6
Topical use, acute conditions	6	200	6	10	333	10

Aromatic Baths

From Egypt to India, the ancients had elaborate ritual ablutions that were combinations of hot and cold baths, ointments, and aromatic massages. Essential oils and baths have synergistic effects. Essential oils enhance the pleasure of the bath and, to quote Robert Tisserand, "If they please the nose, they also please the spirit. Then there is the physiological action of the essences on the nervous system and the rest of the body" (*Aromatherapy to Heal and Tend the Body*, 1989).

Dosage for Aromatic Baths

Aromatic baths are generally very safe provided that the essential oils are properly dispersed into the water. Essential oils do not mix with water. Therefore, it is always recommended to use a dispersant whenever using essential oils in a bath.

You can use an unscented liquid soap or foaming bath gel, a base for bath oil (we recommend a nonfoaming dispersible base), or unscented bath salts or crystals. Aroma Véra produces four unscented bases that are suitable for making an aromatic bath: unscented bath and shower gel, unscented bath salt, unscented bath oil, and an emulsifier. An emulsifier is a product that allows the dispersion of essential oils in water. I strongly recommend using a dispersant for your bath preparations to avoid possible skin irritations. The recommended dose for a full bath is ten to fifteen drops of essential oils. The maximum dose is three drops per bath; see Table 13.

Aromatic Body Wrap

- Lay a blanket on a comfortable horizontal surface (bed, carpet, massage table, etc.).
- Cover the blanket with a plastic foil and place a large towel on top.
- In a spray bottle, mix ten to fifteen drops of the appropriate blend of essential oils with eight to twelve ounces (200 to 300 milliliters) of hot water and fifty to sixty drops of an emulsifier. (Aroma Véra offers blends of essential oils in an emulsifier that allows an easier and faster dispersion of the oils in the water.)

Table 13
Recommended Oils for Bath and Massage

Purpose	Essential oils	Suggested formula*		Effect
		Oil	No. of drops	
Relaxation/ stress relief	Marjoram, orange, lavender, chamomile, tangerine, spikenard, neroli, ylang-ylang	Lavender Tangerine Marjoram Chamomile ✓	3 3 3 1	Will induce a deep relaxation of the tissues, muscles, and joints, and reestablish a good balance of energy
Energy/ tissue firming	Lemon, peppermint, sage, thyme, rosemary, ginger, nutmeg, pepper	Peppermint Rosemary Ginger	4 3 3	General tonic of the endocrine glands and nervous system; tones the tissue (energetic massage)
Pain Relief, sport massage, arthritis	Birch, rosemary, lavender, thyme, pine chamomile, peppermint, camphor, juniper, ginger, nutmeg	Birch Rosemary Juniper Ginger	5 3 2 2	Rheumatic crisis, neuralgia, sores, and muscular aches
Circulation problems, cellulitis, water retention, obesity	Cypress, geranium, lemon, thyme, grapefruit, juniper, angelica, fennel, birch	Grapefruit Lemon Juniper Cypress Red thyme	4 3 2 2 1	Strengthen the circulatory system (lymphatic system, capillaries, veins) and fluidize the blood; varicosis, hemorrhoids, obesity
Aphrodisiac	Jasmine, ylang-ylang, michelia flowers, cedarwood, geranium, vetiver, clary sage, pepper, cistus, sandalwood, patchouli	Ylang-ylang Jasmine Michelia flowers Sandalwood Patchouli	3 2 2 2 1	A delightful prelude or interlude
Nervousness	Mugwort, petitgrain, marjoram, neroli, rose, spikenard	Neroli Petitgrain Marjoram Spikenard	3 3 3 1	

*For one bath or to prepare 1 ounce (30 milliliters) of massage oil.

♦ Shake well. Spray oil mixture on the towel, shaking constantly. Lie on the towel and wrap it around your whole body. Wrap the plastic foil and the blanket around you.

♦ Breathe, relax, enjoy. . . . Enhance the experience with a quiet room, dim light, and nice, peaceful music.

Body wraps may also be done in "zones" or chakras. Soft cotton bandages are soaked in a bowl of hot water with ten to fifteen drops of essential oil blend, and the body is wrapped in sections. You can apply different oils on different parts of the body, one for each zone or body part. For instance, you could apply detoxifying oils on the lower body to activate toxins elimination and fight cellulitis and relaxing oils on upper back and shoulders where stress and tension tend to accumulate.

Dosage for Aromatic Body Wrap

Body wraps are a very safe way to apply essential oils. We strongly recommend the use of an emulsifier to ensure proper dispersion of the essential oils. The recommended dose for a full body wrap is ten to fifteen drops. Maximum dose is fifty drops. The same cautions apply to body wraps as to massages (no ketones and only low doses of phenols). The most effective treatment is to follow the body wrap with a massage using the same blends.

Salt Glow

The salt glow (also called body gommage) is an exfoliating and detoxifying treatment that is very popular in Europe and

Asia, especially Korea and Japan. For a body gommage treatment, mix one ounce of finely ground sea salt with ten to fifteen drops of essential oils (cypress, thyme, grapefruit, lemon, juniper, angelica, fennel). Moisten the salt with water or mix with a carrier oil or unscented lotion to obtain a paste that can be spread easily. Apply the preparation with your fingertips or with a washcloth or a loofa. Apply with circular movement on the entire body, especially hips and thighs. A body gommage exfoliates dead cells from the outer skin layer, deep cleanses the pores, activates capillary and lymphatic circulation, and stimulates the elimination of toxins. It is excellent for cellulitis or weight problems and can be done at home before the morning shower or before a bath. I recommend doing this two to three times a week.

SKIN CARE USES OF ESSENTIAL OILS

Applied to the skin, essential oils regulate the activity of the capillaries and restore vitality to the tissues. According to Marguerite Maury (*The Secret of Life and Youth*), they are natural rejuvenating agents. They facilitate the elimination of waste matter and dead cells and promote the regeneration of new, healthy cells (cytophylactic power).

The most pleasant scents (especially flower oils) are the most useful for skin care. They can be used in facial steam baths, compresses, masks, and body wraps. They can be added to any kind of lotion, skin cream, gel, toilet water, or perfume. As a rule, never apply essential oils undiluted on the skin.

Floral waters are particularly well suited to skin care. Milder and easier to use than essential oils, they are recommended for sensitive and inflamed skins. Essential oils and floral water have more or less the same indications. You can use plain floral water for compresses. You should use floral water instead of water in any skin care preparation. Finally, you will get an excellent facial tonic and astringent using floral water with a spray bottle (rose, sage, rosemary, lavender, cypress, etc.)—very refreshing. Floral waters retain the water-soluble plant chemicals, which do not appear in the finished essential oil. See Table 14 for a guide to oils for specific facial applications.

Facial Steam Bath

Add five to fifteen drops of oils to a bowl of hot water. Drape a large towel over your head and lower your face into the steam, letting it unclog your pores. Add a few drops every five minutes (ten to fifteen minutes total).

Facial Compresses

Add five drops of the appropriate blend of oils to a bowl of warm water; soak cotton or cloth. Apply on your face for five minutes. Resoak and reapply up to three times (recommended dose, five drops; maximum dose, ten drops). Avoid phenolic oils.

Eye Compresses

Use cotton pads soaked in warm floral water. For puffiness, irritation, and most eye compresses use chamomile floral water. For wrinkles around the eyes, use rose floral waters.

Masks

Facial masks are cleansing, nourishing, and revitalizing; they promote the elimination of waste material and stimulate local blood circulation. They can be soothing and moisturizing, depending on the ingredients. We strongly recommend using an emulsifier to ensure proper dispersion of the oils. Basic ingredients for a mask are clay, oatmeal, fruit or vegetable pulp, vegetable oil, floral water, and essential oils.

♦ Put a few spoonfuls of clay and soaked oatmeal in a bowl; add the fruit (or vegetable) pulp and juice, a teaspoon of vegetable oil (wheat germ for instance), and five drops of essential oils.
♦ Stir, then add floral water, herb tea, or plain water until the mixture has the right consistency.
♦ Apply to your face with your fingertips and let mask dry for up to fifteen minutes, then gently remove it with a wet sponge.
♦ Apply floral water to close the pores.
♦ Normal skin needs a mask every one to two weeks.

The recommended dose is five drops in a mask, with fifteen drops being the maximum dose. In addition to oatmeal, clay, essential oils, and floral water, you can use:

For acne: cabbage, grape, yeast.
For oily skin: cabbage, cucumber, lemon, grape, pear, strawberry.
For dry skin: melon, carrot, avocado, wheat germ oil.
For sensitive skin: honey, apple, grape, melon.
For mature skin: apple, avocado, wheat germ oil.
For normal skin: avocado, lemon, peach, wheat germ oil.

Caution: Avoid phenolic oils, use only small amounts of green clay on dry skin, and use only small amounts of seaweed on sensitive skin.

Facial Oils

Facial oils can be used for facial massage, or they can be used as moisturizer, nourisher, and protectant at the end of a skin care session. For a facial massage, we recommend using a base of sweet almond oil or hazelnut oil. For a facial nourishment, to use at the end of the skin care session, we recommend hazelnut oil (90

Table 14
Essential Oils for Skin Care

Skin type/ problem	Essential oils
Normal skin	Clary sage, geranium, lavender, ylang-ylang, rosewood
Dry skin	*Sage lavandulifolia,* clary sage, cedarwood, sandalwood, rose, palmarosa, carrot
Oily skin	Lavender, lemon, geranium, basil, camphor, frankincense, rosemary, ylang-ylang
Inflamed skin	German chamomile, helycrisum, clary sage, lavender, myrrh, patchouli, carrot, floral waters
Sensitive skin	Roman chamomile, neroli, rosewood, floral waters
Acne	Cajeput, tea tree, eucalyptus, juniper, lavender, palmarosa, niaouli
Eczema	Cedarwood, German chamomile, lavender, sage, patchouli, rose, benzoin
Rejuvenation	Benzoin, frankincense, sandalwood, cedarwood, geranium, lavender, myrrh, rosemary, carrot
Seborrhea	Bergamot, lavender, *sage lavandulifolia,* cypress, patchouli
Broken capillaries	Rose, ylang-ylang
Wrinkles	Fennel, lemon, palmarosa, myrrh, frankincense, patchouli, clary sage, carrot

percent) with vitamin E (2 percent), evening primrose oil (4 percent), and borage oil (4 percent) blended together.

Dosage

The recommended concentration for facial oils is 3 to 4 percent, or thirty to forty drops in one ounce (thirty milliliters) of carrier. The maximum concentration is 8 percent or eighty drops in one ounce (thirty milliliters) of carrier oil.

Suggested Base for a Facial Oil (One-Ounce or Thirty-Milliliter Preparation)

Hazelnut oil: 8 ml
Squalene: 8 ml
Jojoba: 8 ml
Helio-carrot: 3 ml
Evening primrose, borage, or rosa mosceta (or a combination of the three): 2 ml
Vitamin E: 1 ml

Caution for Use of Essential Oils in Skin Care

General Cautions

- As a general rule, never apply pure essential oils directly to the face.
- Never use essential oils around the eyes.
- Avoid using phenolic oils on the face (clove, oregano, savory, red thyme).
- In sunny climates, do not use bergamot oil, and use only low concentrations of citrus oils (lemon, lime, orange, tangerine). All citrus oils, especially bergamot, increase photo-

synthesis and may cause sunspots.
- On dry skin, do not use phenolic or drying oils, such as eucalyptus or the oils rich in terpenes (pine and fir).
- On inflamed and sensitive skin, lower essential oils concentration, and do not use phenolic oils.

Lotions, Potions, Body Oils, Bath Oils, Ointments

Numerous stories of scented ointments or potions, from the remotest antiquity to the Renaissance, from the holy Bible to the most lascivious oriental tales, are recounted. For example, Mary Magdalene gave a foot rub to Christ with precious ointments, and according to venomous tongues, Cleopatra owed her seductive power to her secret potions rather than to her beauty. Lotions, potions, creams, and ointments would have the following basic ingredients:

16 A solidifier (lanolin or beeswax)
An oil (sweet, almond, avocado, olive, coco—refer to section on massage oil vegetable oil with recommendations for your type of skin)
Distillates or flower water (or distilled water)
A blend of essential oils (see "skin care")

The kind of product you create will depend on the proportion of the ingredients (for a cream use 1 ounce beeswax, 4 ounces vegetable oil, 2 ounces water, 1/4 ounce essential oils). Melt the solidifier in a double saucepan, and slowly add the oil and water, stirring continuously. Let the mixture cool a bit until it starts to thicken, then add the essential oils and stir thoroughly. Store in tightly closed opaque jars.

Hair Care

Mix ¼ ounce of essential oil in 16 ounces of a good shampoo or hair conditioner.

Scalp rub: Flower waters or ¼ ounce essential oils in 4 ounces grain alcohol or sweet almond oil
Dry hair: Cade, cedarwood
Hair loss: Cedarwood, juniper, lavender, rosemary, sage
Normal hair: Chamomile, lavender, ylang-ylang
Oily hair: Lemongrass, rosemary

Scalp diseases: Cedarwood, rosemary, sage, cade
Dandruff: Rosemary, cedarwood, cade

SAFETY GUIDELINES

1 drop = 1 oz herb

Essential oils are very powerful substances that should be treated with respect; they are highly concentrated plant extracts and should not be abused. Each drop is equivalent to at least one ounce of plant material. Therefore, it is always important to carefully respect the doses (see Table 15). In most cases, essential oils are more potent in infinitesimal doses. Increasing the dosage will not usually increase efficacy.

Table 15
Recommended Dosages for the Use of Essential Oils

Application	%	Drops in			Milliliters in	Use
		1 oz	2 oz	4 oz	100 ml	
Massage						
Full body massage	1.50	15	30	60	1.50	15 ml (½ oz) for full body
Local massage	3.00	30	60	120	3.00	10 to 15 drops on area
Topical application	6.00	60	120	240	6.00	5 drops on point
Bath						
Foaming bath gel	3.00	30	60	120	3.00	15 ml (½ oz) in one bath
Bath oil	5.00	50	100	200	5.00	10 ml (⅓ oz) in one bath
Bath salts and crystals	3.00	30	60	120	3.00	15 ml (½ oz) in one bath
Skin						
Facial sauna						5 to 10 drops in hot water
Compresses						5 to 10 drops in warm water
Mask	2.00	20	40	80	2.00	10 g (⅓ oz) per mask
Face oil	2.00	20	40	80	2.00	3 to 5 drops for facial massage

Some oils, such as the phenolic oils, can be irritating, while others, like the ketones, can be toxic. Proper dosage is critical. The recommended dosage for each type of application and the maximum dosage for safe use are listed in Table 15.

CONCLUSION

When you first step into the essential world, you might be a little bit surprised, or even slightly turned off. Your olfactory system will have to be reeducated, or rather detoxified. After years of neglect and abuse with junk perfumes, your nose might not be able to fully appreciate the richness of natural fragrances. Just like when you change your eating habits from junk food to a more healthy diet, you cannot really appreciate the full flavor of a lettuce leaf, a plain radish, or a bowl of brown rice. But when you start to detoxify, your taste greatly improves and refines, and soon you do not want to come back to junk again.

Then the power of fragrances moves you every day; you play with them, dance with them, create with them. They connect you to the quintessence of the realm of plants and will "make thee glad, merry, gracious and well-beloved of all men."

SEVEN

The Essential Oils

Plants are classified in botanical families according to the structure of their flowers. This classification goes beyond the flower itself, and each plant of the same family appears like a variation of the basic model of the type: same leaf and seed structure, similar rhythm (in space and time), and similar chemical composition.

With Goethe, the anthroposophists believe in an archetypal plant that exhibits the structural potentialities of the vegetable kingdom and manifests itself through different degrees of differentiation in families, species, and chemotypes. In this system, each type expressed by the botanical families represents a certain degree of evolution of the archetypal model—a certain level of actualization of its potentialities, from the primitive equisetaceáe (horsetail) to the most evolved rosaceae (rose, apple, etc.). Differentiation of the type generates the species (or genus), which is then further differentiated in subspe-

cies and chemotypes. In the anthroposophic vision, inspired by the works of Paracelsus and the study of homeopathy, the physical aspect of the plants and the nature of their interactions with the environment are correlated with their medicinal properties. A type of therapeutic activity is attributed to each botanical family, variations being related to each plant of the family. This approach is quite rich and accurate. It is fairly consistent with the more classical systems of herbal therapy and aromatherapy: there are some obvious similarities between the recommended uses of plants in the same family.

While a wildcrafter in southern France, I experienced the accuracy of such a vision. In some powerful experiences of intimate communication with plants, I felt that the plants introduced themselves to me and I could tell the medicinal properties or even the names of plants that I had never seen before. More generally, I found that careful observation of the plant and its environment told me much about its activity.

At any rate, classification of essential oils by botanical families tells more about their therapeutic activity than a mere alphabetical classification, and that will be my approach to this chapter. I hope that this gives my readers a better understanding of aromatherapy.

SYNTHETICS VERSUS NATURAL: DOES IT MAKE SCENTS?

Many people think that molecules produced through the processes of life are more active in a living context (such as medicine) than their synthetic counterparts are, although they cannot really be chemically differentiated from their natural cousins. There is even growing evidence that this belief is well founded. Along the same line of thought, a natural extract is often found to be more efficient than its main active ingredient.

Is it possible that molecules have some kind of memory? That they store the information pertaining to their history? That life shares a common pool of memories? That natural molecules are more accurate in dealing with living organisms because they have stored living memory? If so, a natural molecule could "know" how to deal with other living molecules. Each molecule belonging to a given extract would have a memory of its companions and could predictably be more efficient when not separated from these companions.

THE CONCEPT OF MORPHOGENETIC FIELDS

When bicycles were first invented, it took people months to learn how to ride them. How long did it take your kids to learn how to ride their bikes? A few hours? Two days? When the first cars were invented, most people were too scared to even think about driving them. Now the average teenager learns how to drive in very little time. When Einstein introduced the theory of relativity, years passed before a handful of people could figure it out. Currently, relativity is taught in college. How long did it take you to learn how to use a computer? How long did it take your kids? When you look at up-to-date college textbooks, how often do you feel that you haven't any clue to what they are all about?

According to Rupert Sheldrake, all these phenomena can be accounted for by the concept of morphogenetic fields, a theory that we can manifest what we create in our thoughts just by envisioning. To put it simply, a morphogenetic field can be viewed as a landscape, with mountains, valleys, plains, riverbeds, and so on. Each valley, each riverbed corresponds to flows of information, all interconnected. A totally new input of information can be viewed as a small furrow being traced somewhere in the landscape. The more this information is used, the deeper its furrow becomes, and the more likely it will be to attract new information, until it resembles a valley or a main stream. Learning a new technique, for instance, deepens the corresponding furrow. The more people learn this technique, the deeper the furrow, and the easier it becomes for other people to learn the technique.

Of course, a new furrow is generated only when the landscape is ready for it. This would account for the fact that very often, whenever the ground is ready for a new discovery, several people will make this discovery at the same time.* Conversely, whenever an area of the morphogenetic field does not flow, it becomes locally stagnant, and sediment accumulates. Thus, valleys are filled up, riverbeds disappear, and information is buried because of disuse.

The concept of the morphogenetic field is an excellent tool for describing all the processes of evolution, whether evolution of the universe, evolution of species, cultural evolution, or personal evolution. It helps us understand how patterns are created. For example, positive thinking is a personal application of the morphogenetic field; it can act as the path to achieving one's goals by attracting positive experience. The more we imagine ourselves achieving success, the more successful we become. This is why I am an incurable optimist and why I think that pessimists are always wrong especially when they are right.

Botanical families can be viewed as deep valleys in the vegetal morphogenetic field, dividing into the rivers of species and the streams of subspecies of chemotypes. Each of these valleys, rivers, and streams has been generated throughout the ages in close interaction with the local and global environment (other families and species and the ecosystems supporting them, including microorganisms, animals, and humans).

We can see how the concept of the morphogenetic field is in total agreement with the Gaia hypothesis. Our planet is a living organism. Humanity has brought consciousness to this organism—for a purpose, undoubtedly. This purpose cannot be the destruction of the planet. As conscious cells of this organism, we have a responsibility to take care of our planet. Otherwise, we behave like a virus in a sick body, and the organism will try to get ride of us. A lose–lose situation.

Our planet, the body we all live in together, is presently going through an acute toxic crisis. For those of you familiar with natural healing, this means that our planet will most probably need to go through a dramatic discharge process. But this is an emergency. No economic or other consideration can prevail against this absolute necessity. There is now an enormous worldwide awareness of this crisis. This can be viewed as a natural defense mechanism of our planet. We must capitalize on this movement and start acting now. We can do it, individually and collectively.

---

* Interestingly enough, in the late 1970s, my research in logic and the theory of information came very close to the ideas that Rupert Sheldrake was developing (I talked about field of forms; he talks about morphogenetic fields). I presented a paper at the University of California at Berkeley in 1980 to explain my theories. I was not aware of Sheldrake at that time, nor was he aware of my work.

BACK TO THE BOTANICAL FAMILIES

Botanical Families and the Gaia Hypothesis

The vegetable kingdom appeared on our planet long before the animal kingdom. Through evolution, from the primitive moss or fern, it gradually differentiated to generate the thousands of species that we now know. This evolution was at first independent of the animal kingdom (but maybe it was preparing the ground for it—by producing oxygen, for instance). Then, when the first animals appeared on our planet (and they appeared because the morphogenetic field was ready for them), the two realms evolved in close interaction. For example, more and more vegetable species came to depend on insects for pollination. And, of course, animals were totally dependent on plants for their subsistence.

It is not unreasonable to think that this interaction went very far; plants were not only food for the animal kingdom but were also medicine. Animals provided fertilizers; they carried the seeds and buried them, moved the ground with their feet, and trimmed the bushes. If the Gaia hypothesis is well founded—and I believe it is—and if our planet can be viewed as a living organism, this is not surprising.

Certain plants became specialized in their interaction with the animal kingdom. Human intervention further accentuated this process; the plants that are now cultivated domestically have been "created" through a long selection process.

The varieties of corn, wheat, apples, or potatoes that we buy in our supermarkets do not exist in the wild—they were produced through genetic breeding.

The study of botanical families, by going from the global (the vegetable kingdom) to the particular (the species and the subspecies) through the differentiation process (the botanical families), gives us a better understanding of and appreciation for our living planet. Each plant has accumulated through the millions of years of its history the living memory of the vegetable kingdom, the memory of its family, the memory of its genus and its species. All this information is here for us to share and respect. This is an ongoing miracle.

The Plant's Domain of Creativity

When we look at a planet from the perspective of the botanical family, we can learn a lot from the family itself. We also can learn from the part of the plant where its creativity is the most developed, and, in studying aromatherapy, where its essential oil is produced.

Each family seems to have a privileged domain of creativity. The Labiatae and Myrtacea produce their essential oils mostly in the leaves, while the rose produces them in the flower; the citruses in the flower, the fruit, and the leaves; the burseraceae in their exudate; and so on.

Evolution Involution

Each plant goes from the physical sphere, with the germ and then the roots, through the vital sphere with the leaves, and to the astral sphere with the flower in a natural evolution process. It then creates its fruit or seed in an involution back to the physical world.

Essential oils produced in the roots (angelica, vetiver) tend to have a very grounding energy; they have a foodlike quality to them. They are not very refined, but they usually are potent stimulants of the vital functions (especially digestion) of the organism. Typically, they are recommended for anemia.

The plant's leaf system corresponds to its vital body. Essential oils produced in the leaves (eucalyptus, niaouli, peppermint, etc.) have a strong affinity with the prajna energy, the respiratory system. They tone the vital body. Excessive development of the leaf system of a plant is a sign of etheric imbalance that can produce toxicity (as in some Umbelliferae).

The flower is the plant's ultimate achievement. Only the most spiritually evolved plants (such as the rose) can fully create at this level. The production of fragrance is then a sign of intense astral activity. Although the essential oils are found in extremely small amounts in the flowers, their fragrances are typically very intense, although refined in nature. The plants with the most intense floral creativity rarely produce any significant fruit or seed. These plants' creativity is exhausted with the fragrance, and their creation does not belong to the physical plant any longer. Such fragrances have a tendency to be exhilarating (jasmine) or even intoxicating (narcissus).

The essential oils of flowers are then usually very refined and subtle but very hard to extract. They often are too far removed from the physical sphere to be extracted through steam distillation. (Neroli and rose are an exception, as they are particularly well-balanced plants; they both produce edible fruits: oranges and rose hips, respectively) Very sensitive to temperature, their molecules break apart when exposed to heat. Some of them can be extracted by solvents (jasmine, tuberose, narcissus).

The oils produced in the seed bring us back fully into the physical world, being less sophisticated, more humble, and straightforward (citrus fruits, anise, fennel, coriander). They are invigorating and fortifying and show a strong affinity with the digestive system (especially those seeds that are food or spices).

Trees and bushes also have the ability to create oils in their wood (sandalwood, cedarwood). Such oils are centering and equilibrating. Here the creative process is drawn into the heart of the wood. These oils have the power to open our consciousness to high spheres without making us lose control. They are particularly suited to rituals, meditation, and yoga.

Finally, many trees and bushes (myrrh, frankincense, conifers, cistus) produce odorous resins or gums. These essential oils have a strong affinity for the glandular system; they control secretions and demonstrate cosmetic and healing properties (skin care, wounds, ulcers).

EIGHT

Essential Oils in
Botanical Families

Birch (*Betula lenta* and *B. nigra*, Betulaceae)

♦ Traditionally produced in the northeastern United States.
♦ Distillation of the bark: The oil is clear to yellowish.
♦ Fragrance: Balsamic, sweet, warm.
♦ Used in liniments and unguents for muscular and articular aches.

Birch oil contains up to 98% methyl salicylate and therefore is quite often adulterated with the latter product. Two varieties of birch oil have been differentiated: northern birch oils, produced in Pennsylvania, Vermont, and New Hampshire (which apparently is no longer produced), and southern birch oil, produced in the southern part of the Appalachian mountains.

Wintergreen oil is similar to birch oil in its composition; however, it is no longer produced. Therefore, everything sold as wintergreen is either methyl salicylate or birch oil.

Organs: Kidneys, joints.
Medicinal properties: Diuretic; analgesic; purifying, draining (lymphatic), cleansing.
Indications: Rheumatism, arthritis, muscular and articular pains (one of the best remedies); kidney and urinary tract disorders (cystitis, stones, mucus discharge, dropsy); autointoxication caused by poor elimination of urea, cholesterol, glucose; skin diseases.

Burseraceae: Dry Fire

The essential oils of this family include elemi, frankincense, and myrrh. Burseraceae grow in desert tropical areas where the intense cosmic activity promotes the formation of gum and etheric oils. Boswellia (myrrh, frankincense), the most characteristic representatives of the type, grow in the Arabian peninsula, in the most extreme climate of the planet. They are surrounded by a thin cloud of essential oils, which filters the heal w/ formation of scar

sun's rays and freshens the air around them—hence their strong anti-inflammatory action. Burseraceae act against inner fire in the body (bronchitis, cough, pleuristy, phthisis, consumption).

The gum oozes from the incisions of natural fissures in the bark or the wood. It is cicatrizant and vulnerary and has powerful healing properties. It is especially useful in diseases related to secretion (inflammation of the breast or the uterus).

Putrefaction cannot take place in the desert; the air is too dry and the heat too intense. Burseraceae condense the desert energy and therefore have strong antiputrescent effects on corpses. They have a salutary action on ulcers, gangrene, and gastric and intestinal fermentation. The desert is also the place where those who want to go beyond the mundane and superfluous find an austere but powerful environ. There, everything is reduced to essentials. The contemplation of the endless petrified waves of the sandy dunes inspires one to go beyond the always-changing waves of one's own mind and connect with bare infinity and eternity. The powerful comforting scent of myrrh or frankincense carried by the burning wind of the desert gently soothes one's deepest wounds and gives one further inspiration in meditation.

Since antiquity, myrrh and frankincense have been extensively used in incense in rituals and religious ceremonies. They have a very pronounced soothing, comforting, fortifying, and elevating action on the soul and the spirit.

Type of action: Cooling, drying, fortifying.

Domain of action: Skin, lungs, secretion, mind, psychic centers.

Indications: Inflammation (skin, lungs, breast, uterus).

Elemi (Canarium luzonicum)

♦ The gum is produced in the Philippines, Central America, and Brazil.
♦ Distillation of the gum: The oil is colorless to slightly yellow.
♦ Fragrance: Pleasant, balsamic—resembling camphor—and incense-like.
♦ Used in perfumery and in some medical preparations.

Introduced in Europe in the fifteenth century, elemi was an ingredient in numerous balms, unguents, and liniments. It is still used in the balm of Fioraventi and other vulnerary preparations.

Medicinal properties and indications: Similar to those of myrrh and frankincense.

Frankincense (Boswellia carteri)

♦ The gum is produced in northeast Africa and southeast Arabia (Somalia, Ethiopia, Yemen); the supply has been quite erratic lately, because of the political confusion in these countries.
♦ Distillation of the gum: The oil is clear or yellow.
♦ Fragrance: Characteristic—balsamic, camphor-like, spicy, woody, slightly lemony.

♦ Used in cosmetics and perfumery; blends well with almost any scent; makes a good fixative.

One of the most highly priced substances of the ancient world, frankincense was once as valuable as gold. Its trade was one of the major economic activities in some Arabic countries, and its control provoked many local wars. The Queen of Sabah, a main producer of that time, undertook a perilous journey from Somalia to Israel and visited King Solomon to secure the flourishing trade. Frankincense has been burned in temples since antiquity, especially by the Egyptians and the Hebrews; it is still used in the rites of some churches. Frankincense gum was traditionally used to fumigate sick persons to drive out the evil spirits causing the sickness. The Egyptians used it in their rejuvenating unguents.

Medicinal properties and indications: Similar to those of myrrh; special action on breast inflammations and uterine disorders; pregnancy, birth preparation.

Myrrh (Commiphora myrrha)

♦ The gum is produced in the same areas as frankincense, as well as in Libya and Iran.
♦ Distillation of the gum: The oil is yellow to reddish-brown and more or less fluid.
♦ Fragrance: Pleasant, balsamic, camphor-like, musty, incense-like.
♦ Used in perfumery and cosmetics; blends well with many oils; makes a good fixative.

The history of myrrh is closely tied to that of frankincense. These two substances were among the precious drugs reserved for fumigations, embalming, unctions, and liturgical practices. The Egyptian papyrus, the Vedas, the Bible, and the Koran mention the numerous uses of myrrh in ceremonies, in perfumery, and in medicine. Myrrh was an ingredient of many unguents, elixirs, and other multipurpose antidotes.

Medicinal properties: Balsamic, expectorant; astringent, resolutive; anti-inflammatory, antiseptic, antiputrescent, vulnerary, cicatrizant; affects mucous membrane; stimulant, tonic; sedative.

Indications: Inflammation (breast, lungs, gangrene, infected wounds, ulcers); catarrhal conditions (head, lungs, stomach, intestines); tuberculosis, phthisis, bronchitis, cough; hemorrhages (uterine, pulmonary); pregnancy, childbirth.

Cinnamon (Cinnamomum zeylanicum; Lauraceae)

wasting diseases

♦ Produced in Ceylon (the best quality), India, and China.
♦ Distillation of the bark: The oil is reddish-brown. The leaves are also distilled, but the quality of their oil is much lower.
♦ Fragrance: Characteristically spicy, burning.
♦ Widely used in food industry, pharmacy, cosmetics, perfumery.

Certainly one of the oldest spices known, it was already the object of an important trade between India, China, and Egypt more than 4000 years ago. In 2700 B.C., the Chinese emperor Shen Nung call it "kwei" in his pharmacopeia. Cinnamon is often mentioned in the Bible. Yahweh ordered Moses to use it in the fabrication of the holy ointment. It was one of the most important drugs of the Greek and Roman pharmacopeia and was quite renowned for its stomachic, diuretic, tonic, and antiseptic properties.

Medicinal properties: Stimulant (circulatory, cardiac, and pulmonary functions); antiseptic, antiputrescent; antispasmodic; aphrodisiac; parasiticide; irritant and convulsive in high doses.

Indications: Flu, asthenia; spasms, intestinal infections; impotence; childbirth, labor (increase contractions).

Cistus (*Cistus ladaniferus*; Cistaceae)

♦ Produced in Spain and Cyprus.
♦ Distillation of the branches: The oil is reddish-brown.
♦ Fragrance: Musky, balsamic.
♦ Used in expensive perfumes because it makes a good fixative and gives a natural musk note to the blends.

Cistus, or rock rose, is a small bush growing in dry rocky areas of the Mediterranean countries, especially in Crete and Cyprus. Its leaves naturally exude gum called labdanum. This gum has been highly appreciated in perfumery, cosmetics, and medicine since antiquity and was one of the ingredients of the "holy ointment" of the Bible.

The gum sticks to the wool of sheep grazing on the hills as they walk through the bushes, so shepherds in Crete and Cyprus used to comb the wool of their sheep to collect the precious gum. Labdanum was also collected by whipping the bushes with a special whip, this method giving a much better quality. Unfortunately, both methods have now been abandoned, and labdanum is not produced any more.

Medicinal properties: Tonic, astringent; nervous sedative, antispasmodic; vulnerary.

Indications: Diarrhea, dysentery, intestinal troubles; nervousness, insomnia; ulcers.

Compositae: Realization, Organization, and Structure

Essential oils of this family include chamomile, everlasting, mugwort, and tarragon. Other oils of interest are arnica, calendula, tansy, yarrow, wormwood. The compositae are characterized by their inflorescence, a collection of small flowers forming a unique superior entity. This basic simple structure is able to generate such a diversity that, with about eight hundred genera and thirteen thousand species, the compositae constitute the largest botanical family.

Unlike orchids, another large family with amazing floral variations, Compositae grow all over the world in large settlements. They live in almost every terrestrial zone, except the far north and the tropical forest, from seashores to mountain tops, from desert to swamps, with a preference for open spaces widely exposed to light such as meadows and steppes.

Very adaptive and intensely associated with light, Compositae live primarily in the floral sphere. Because they embody a perfect balance of etheric and astral forces, the therapeutic activity of the plants of this family shows great diversity.

Chamomile (Anthemis nobilis, A. mixta, Chamomilla matricaria, Ormenis multicolis)

Roman

stimulant of leukocytes

♦ Produced in France, Morocco, Spain, Egypt.
♦ Distillation of flowers: The oil of *Anthemis nobilis* (Roman chamomile) and *Anthemis mixta* is yellow, while the oils of *Chamomilla matricaria* is light blue and *Ormenis multicolis* (blue chamomile) is dark blue, owing to the presence of azulene.
♦ Fragrance: Refreshing, aromatic.
♦ Used in perfumery, cosmetics, and pharmacy.

Dedicated to the sun by the Egyptians for its febrifuge properties, chamomile is probably one of the oldest known medicinal plants. It was regarded as the plant's physician and was thought to keep other plants in good health.

Interest in chamomile has recently been revived with the discovery of azulene, an excellent anti-inflammatory agent, which is not present in the fresh flower but is formed when the plant is distilled. Many different botanical species around the world are called chamomile. Roman chamomile (*Anthemic nobilis*) and German chamomile (*Chamomilla matricaria*) are the most commonly used in herbology. The oil called chamomile mixta or "wild chamomile" is distilled from the wild in southern Spain and Morocco. Blue chamomile is distilled in Morocco and Egypt. A pineapple-scented chamomile grows throughout the United States (and has not been distilled as far as I know). Other varieties of chamomile grow in different parts of the world but are used only locally.

Roman chamomile is an excellent calming and soothing oil and a liver stimulant. Matricaria (its German name means "mother herb") is especially indicated for female disorders. See also the essential oil quick reference charts for the differences between the chamomiles.

Matricaria is especially recommended for feminine diseases (painful or irregular period, excessive loss of blood, hemorrhage). The whole plant is aerial, radiant; each beam terminates in a white and gold flower with a bulging receptacle, which encloses a drop of air. This flower manifests a subdued ardor, an appeased and soothing flame.

Chamomile likes light; it grows on roadsides and in open fields, in light sandy soils. Its affinity for the air element and its particular connection with the aerial spheres indicate the strong therapeutic action of chamomile on the abnormal astral processes in the human organism. It is beneficent against spasms, convulsions, hypersensitivity, menstruation troubles, colic, and neuralgic aches.

Medicinal properties: Anti-inflammatory (especially matricaria), antispasmodic, mild nervous sedative (children), anticonvulsive, antidepressant; emmena-

sweat

counter inflammatio

gogue; antianemic; febrifuge, sudorific; hepatic, cholagogue; antiseptic; analgesic; stimulant of leukocytosis; cicatrizant, vulnerary; local vasoconstrictor.

Indications: Infectious diseases, fever; anemia; inflammation; migraine, depression, headache, convulsions, insomnia, vertigo, irritability, hysteria; dysmenorrhea, amenorrhea, vaginitis, menopausal problems, vulvar pruritus; liver and spleen congestion; painful digestion, digestive problems of children, gastralgia, gastritis; ulcers (stomach, intestines); colic, colitis; neuralgia, rheumatism; teething pains, toothache, gingivitis; earache; wounds, burns, boils, urticaria, dermatitis, skin diseases, skin care; conjunctivitis; pronounced effect on the mind and nervous system (anger, oversensitiveness, temper tantrums of children).

Everlasting (Helicrysum italicum)

♦ Produced in southern France, Italy, Yugoslavia.
♦ Distillation of the whole plant: The oil is yellowish.
♦ Fragrance: Strongly aromatic.

Everlasting is a fairly new oil in aromatherapy. My friend Gilles Garcin, with whom I used to distill wild lavender in the southern Alps of France, might very well be the first one to have distilled the plant for aromatherapy (incidentally, he used Henri Viaud's distillery). It has proved to be valuable for wounds and bruises.

Medicinal properties: Anti-inflamma-tory, antiphlogistic (according to Kurt Schnaubelt, it is ever more potent than blue chamomile); cell regenerator.

Indications: Hemorrhage; bruises, trauma; open wounds.

Mugwort (Artemisia vulgaris, A. herba alba)

♦ Produced in Morocco and North Africa.
♦ Distillation of the whole plant: The oil is yellowish-brown.
♦ Fragrance: Strongly aromatic, slightly musky.

Named after the goddess Artemis (or Diana), protectress of virgins, mugwort had an ancient reputation as a specific for female cycles. It was also a magical plant, known to increase psychic power.

Organs: Female genitals.

Medicinal properties: Emmenagogue (abortive at high doses), regulator of the feminine cycle; antispasmodic; cholagogue, tonic, aperitive; vermifuge.

Indications: Menstrual troubles (amenorrhea; dismenorrhea; scanty, insufficient, or excessive periods); hysteria, convulsion, epilepsy, nervous vomiting; ascariasis, oxyuriasis.

Tarragon (Artemisia dracunculus)

♦ Produced in France, United States, Belgium.
♦ The oil is obtained by distillation of the plant, almost colorless. The fragrance is anise-y and aromatic.

Medicinal properties: Stimulant of the digestive system (stomach and intestine);

antispasmodic; carminative, aperitive; vermifuge.

Indications: Dyspepsia, hiccup; dystonia, weak digestion; aerophagy, fermentation; intestinal parasites.

Coniferae: The Air Element; Light, Inner Warmth versus Cold; and Verticality

Essential oils of this family include cedarwood, cypress, fir, juniper, pine, spruce, and thuja. Other oils of interest are cade, sabine, therebentine. A wide belt of Coniferae circles the frigid and temperate zones of both hemispheres, from the far north or far south and almost to the mountaintops, depending on altitude. In tropical zones they grow only at high altitudes.

The type is imposing in its simplicity, dominated by a vertical and linear principle. Everything is structured around the central vertical trunk; the trunk is surrounded with branches shaped like small trees, and the leaves are reduced to long needles placed in spirals around the twigs. The floral process is reduced to its minimum: the cone of flowers, a terminal twig surrounded by dense ligneous leaves, bears the nude reproductive organs (stamens or pistil) on the axil of its leaves. The longevity of Coniferae, ruled by Saturn, gives us the oldest and highest trees in the world. In some species, the trunks themselves are virtually immune to rot (prehistoric cypresses found in coal mines in Silesia were used to make furniture!).

The coniferous forest appears immemorial and eternal. Its solemnity, noble majesty, and powerful magnificence bring us back to primordial nature. This forest inspires devotion and respect and opens the heart "to the most ancient, the most basic and primordial feelings of the creation" (Goethe). Troubled souls find rest and strength there.

Coniferae also produce in abundance etheric oils and resins, which fill up the trunks, branches, and needles. In certain species, the resin production is so intense that the trees exude it through their cones or their trunks. Such a phenomenon indicates a deep characteristic relationship between this type and the forces of light and warmth. Because Coniferae live in cold climates, they have to develop an intense inner fire to face the long, rigorous winters until the overflowing light of summer, with its clear nights and its midnight sun. These processes of warmth relate to life and generate substances (essential oils, resins, balms) and are at the origin of the curative power of Coniferae, which is warming and revivifying. Their zone of action is the cold area of the body: the nervous system. The oils of Coniferae are best taken through the lungs (inhalation or aromatic diffuser), where they communicate the *prajna* of the type.

Type of action: Tonic, revivifying, appeasing, warming.

Domain of action: Nervous system, lungs, glandular system.

Indications: Stress, deficiency of the nervous system; lung problems; rheumatism, arthritis.

Cedarwood (*Cedrus atlantica*)

♦ Produced in Morocco.
♦ *Cedrus deodorata* is distilled in the Himalayas. The cedar of Virginia, distilled in the United States, is a juniper (*Juniperus virginiana* and *J. mexicana*); the oil, however, is very similar to real cedarwood oil.
♦ Distillation of the sawdust: The oil is thick and golden-brown, like the color of old gold.
♦ Fragrance: Deep, woody, balsamic, very pleasant, like sandalwood.
♦ Used as a fixative in perfumes; blends well with many oils and gives a woody note to preparations.

Egyptians used cedarwood oil for embalming; it was one of the ingredients of *mithridat,* a famous poison antidote that was used for centuries. One of the most majestic trees, the Lebanese cedar (like its close relative, atlas cedar, growing in Morocco) expresses a great spiritual strength. Egyptians used its wood to build the doors of their temples, where its fragrance would stimulate psychic centers of the worshipers. The effects of cedarwood oil on the mind are similar to those of sandalwood.

Medicinal properties: Antiseptic, fungicidal, antiputrescent; expectorant; stimulant.

Indications: Cystitis, gonorrhea, urinary tract disorders; hair care (hair loss, dandruff, scalp diseases); respiratory conditions; skin disease (eczema, dermatitis, ulcers); anxiety, nervous tension.

Cypress (*Cupressus sempervirens*)

♦ Produced in France, Spain, Morocco.
♦ Distillation of branches: The oil is yellow to brown.
♦ Fragrance: Balsamic, woody, somewhat harsh.

The ancient Egyptians used cypress in their medical preparations; its wood, almost immune to rot, was used to make the sarcophagi for the mummies.

Medicinal properties: Astringent, vasoconstrictor, tonic for the veins; antispasmodic; diuretic, antirheumatic, antisudorific; antiseptic.

Indications: Hemorrhoids, varicose veins; enuresis; whooping cough, asthma; ovary dysfunction (dysmenorrhoea, menopausal problems); perspiration.

Fir (*Abies balsamea*)

♦ Produced in northeast United States and Canada.
♦ Distillation of branches.
♦ Fragrance: Fresh, balsamic, very pleasant; one of the finest coniferous scents.

The fir pine tree exudes a resin called fir balsam that the North American Indians used for medicinal and religious purposes. It was introduced in Europe in the beginning of the seventeenth century, and its action was compared to that of Venetian turpentine, highly valued at the time.

Medicinal properties: Respiratory antiseptic, expectorant; vulnerary.

Indications: Respiratory diseases; genitourinary infections.

пихта – Abies
ель – Picca
лиственница – Larix
сосна – Pinus

resin – смола
наибольшее ... деревьев – сосна

хвойные-семейств
кипарисовых

Juniper (Juniperus communis)

♦ Produced in Yugoslavia, Italy, and France.
♦ Distillation of the berries (gives the best quality) or the small branches: The oil is colorless, yellowish, or pale green.
♦ Fragrance: Terbenthinate, hot, balsamic.

Juniper was burned as incense to ward off evil spirits or to serve as a disinfectant in time of epidemic diseases. Tibetans used it for religious and medicinal purposes. The smallest of coniferae grows in arid and inhospitable areas, where its presence is like a consolation. During Christmas ceremonies in Germany, it represents the tree of life. It hides its rough, bitter fruits in the midst of thick needles; these fruits are salutary for everyone who has abused terrestrial food. It is an excellent diuretic, digestive, and hepatic. Its distorted shape and hard, knotty, twisted wood indicate an obvious affinity with joints, arthritis, and rheumatism. Juniper can influence the effects of old age.

Medicinal properties: Diuretic, antiseptic (urinary tract), antirheumatic, (promotes the elimination of uric acid and toxins); stomachic; antidiabetic. Tonic: nervous system, visceral functions, digestive system; fortifies the memory; rubefacient; vulnerary.

Indications: Urinary tract infections, kidney stones, blennorrhoea, cystitis, oliguria; diabetes; rheumatism, arteriosclerosis; general weariness, nervous fatigue; amenorrhea, dysmenorrhea, painful menstruation; dermatitis, eczema.

Сосна обыкновенная

Pine (Pinus sylvestris)

♦ Distillation of small branches: The oil is colorless.

Produced in the former Soviet Union, Germany, and France, *Pinus maritimus* is distilled in France. Various species closely related to *P. sylvestris* are distilled in Austria, Italy, and Yugoslavia.

Medicinal properties: Expectorant, pulmonary antiseptic; stimulant of adrenocortical glands; hepatic and urinary antiseptic; rubefacient.

Indications: Pulmonary diseases; urinary infections.

ель

Spruce (Picea mariana)

♦ Produced in the same area as fir.
♦ Distillation of branches: The oil is colorless.
♦ Fragrance: Similar to fir, but deeper.

Spruce oil is excellent for balancing the energy. It is recommended for any type of psychic work for its opening and elevating, through grounding, quality. In the diffuser, it is excellent for yoga and meditation.

Medicinal properties and indications: Same as fir.

Thuja (Thuja occidentalis)

highly toxic

♦ Produced in Canada and the United States (Vermont, New Hampshire).

The oil is obtained by distillation of small branches and twigs and has a yellowish color. It is highly toxic and therefore should not be taken internally without the supervision of a medical specialist.

Medicinal properties: Diuretic, urinary sedative; expectorant; antirheumatic; vermifuge.

Indications: Prostatic hypertrophy, cystitis; rheumatism; intestinal parasites; warts.

Geranium (*Pelargonium graveolens* and *P. roseum*, Geraniaceae)

♦ Produced in Reunion, Comoro Islands, Egypt, Morocco.

♦ Distillation of the plant: The oil is greenish-yellow.

♦ Fragrance: Strong, sweet, roselike (almost too strong when it is pure but becomes very pleasant when diluted).

♦ Widely used in perfumery and cosmetics; blends very well with rose, citrus, and almost any oil.

Old herbals mention geranium of Herb Robert (*Geranium robertianum*), which grows wild in the temperate zones of the globe. This plant is totally different from the pelargonium used for the extraction of essential oils. Although they both belong to the same botanical family, their uses are different.

It has been discovered recently that geranium has the power to develop an extremely wide variety of chemotypes, none of them being distilled commercially at this point. The reason for such variations is not yet clear. In fact, geranium can be made to imitate almost any fragrance. In addition to the rose geranium, others—tangerine geranium, lemon geranium, lime geranium, etc.—are found in nurseries. Apparently, the species can produce almost any possible chemotype, including the hot, burning thymols and carvacrols that seem so remote from the sweet-smelling rose geranium that most people know. This seems to indicate a strong adaptability, indicative of immuno-stimulant properties.

Organs: Kidneys.

Medicinal properties: Astringent, hemostatic, cicatrizant, antiseptic; antidiabetic, diuretic; stimulant of adrenal cortex; insect repellent.

Indications: Diabetes, kidney stones; adrenocortical deficiency; tonsillitis, sore throat; hemorrhage; burns, wounds, ulcers; skin disease, skin care; nervous tension, depression.

Ginger (*Zingiber officinale*, Zingiberaceae)

♦ Produced in China, India, Malaysia.

♦ Distillation of the rhizome: The oil is sightly yellow to dark yellow.

♦ Fragrance: Characteristic (camphor-like, aromatic, citrusy).

♦ Widely used in the eastern countries (especially India, China, Japan) in pharmaceutical preparations. Many used in the food and beverage industries.

Ginger has been used for thousands of years in India and China for its remarkable medicinal properties and for its culinary enhancement. It is still one of the major remedies prescribed by macrobiotic therapists and Chinese doctors. Dioscorides recommends it for digestion and stomach weakness. It was mentioned in the Middle Ages as a tonic, stimulant, and febrifuge. It is also an ingredient of the balm of Fioraventi.

Organs: Digestive system.

Medicinal properties: Tonic, stimulant; stomachic, carminative; analgesic; febrifuge; antiscorbutic.

Indications: Deficiency of the digestive system (dyspepsia, flatulence, loss of appetite, etc.); impotence; rheumatic pain.

Graminae: The Nutritious Family

Essential oils of this family include citronella, lemongrass, *Litsea cubeba*, palmarosa, and vetiver. A wide majority of the plants covering the ground belong to the Graminae family. From the poles to the equator, from the swamps to the deserts, this family shows an amazing adaptability and diversity. Its ability to cover almost exclusively huge areas denotes a singular strength. This strength lies in its powerful root system, forming an intricate network that blends almost perfectly with the soil (to create lawns, modern gardeners lay on the soil a kind of carpet that is vegetal and ground together). Above this intense root system, the aerial part of Graminae is dominated by a linear principle: long narrow leaves and straight stems. Even the inflorescence (ear) obeys this principle.

This family does not spend much energy in the floral process—it is entirely dedicated to another aim: Graminae above all is the nutritious family. Its leaves and seeds are a gift to the animal kingdom: grass for herbivores, and grain (wheat, rice, corn, barley, oats) for rodents, birds, and humans.

Graminae has the potential to develop fragrances—like the scent of freshly cut hay! But it usually remains a potential, nascent fragrance. Only under the tropics has this ability been fully developed in some species. The herbs of lemongrass, citronella, *Litsea cubeba*, and palmarosa have a fresh, green, lemony, slightly rosy fragrance. Vetiver produces essential oils in its roots.

Citronella (Cymbopogon nardus)

- ◆ Produced in China, Malaysia, Sri Lanka, Central America.
- ◆ Distillation of the herb: The oil is yellow.
- ◆ Fragrance: Fresh, green, lemony.
- ◆ Widely used in the soap industry, deodorizers, insecticide, sanitary products. Few uses in perfumery. The herb is used in Chinese food.

Medicinal properties and indications: Disinfection of rooms; insecticide.

Lemongrass (Cymbopogon citratus)

- ◆ Produced in India, Central America, and Brazil, *Cymbopogon flexuosus* produces an essential oil also called Indian verbena (not the real essential oil of verbena, which is ten times more expensive).
- ◆ Distillation of the herb: The oil is yellow to reddish-brown.
- ◆ Fragrance: Fresh, lemony, finer than citronella.

♦ Widely used in the soap industry and in perfumery.

According to the Indian pharmacopeia, lemongrass was traditionally used by the Indian as an antidote against infectious diseases, fevers, and cholera.

Medicinal properties: Stimulant of the digestive system (stomachic, carminative, digestive); antiseptic; diuretic; insect repellent.

Indications: Digestive troubles (dyspepsia, colic, flatulence); disinfection, deodorization; pediculosis, scabies.

Veterinary uses: Parasites, digestive troubles.

Litsea cubeba

♦ Produced in China.
♦ Distillation of the herb: The oil is yellow.
♦ Fragrance: Fresh, green, lemony.
♦ Widely used in perfumery and in the soap industry, deodorizers, sanitary products.

Although it is closely related to citronella and lemongrass, *Litsea cubeba* has a much nicer fragrance. It is a fairly new oil in aromatherapy, mostly used for blending (especially in the diffuser). It gives a pleasant, fresh, lemony top note to any blend.

Medicinal properties and indications: Same as lemongrass.

Palmarosa (Cymbopogon martini)

♦ Produced in India, Africa, Comoro Islands, Madagascar.
♦ Distillation of the herb: The oil is yellow.

♦ Fragrance: Fresh, roselike.
♦ Widely used in perfumery and cosmetology (and to adulterate or dilute rose oil, one of the most expensive essential oils).

Medicinal properties: Antiseptic cellular stimulant, hydrating; febrifuge; digestive stimulant.

Indications: Skin care—wrinkles, acne, etc. (reestablishes the physiological balance of the skin, immediate calming and refreshing action); digestive atonia.

Vetiver (Andropogon muricatus)

♦ Produced in Comoro Islands, Caribbean islands, Reunion.
♦ The oil is obtained from the roots: It is deep brown and very thick.
♦ Fragrance: Deep, hearty, woody (slightly reminiscent of tobacco plant or clary), musky, sandalwoodlike.
♦ Used mostly in perfumery and cosmetics; makes a very good fixative.

With vetiver, the aromatic process is drawn into the roots, wherein lies the power of Graminae. Its fragrance is then an actualization in the odoriferous sphere of the potentialities that the type usually expresses in the nutritious sphere. The characteristic earthy, realistic, almost materialistic scent definitively accounts for the nutritious aspect of the family, while the musky note reminds one of its animal connection.

Graminae produce the most sacred food of the vegetable kingdom: wheat, rice, and corn—food beyond food, gift of the gods to the human realm. Vetiver expresses this fundamental aspect of the type through its sandalwoodlike note; it is inspiring and uplifting.

Indication: Arthritis.

Jasmine (*Jasminum officinalis*)

♦ Produced in southern France, North Africa (Egypt, Tunisia, Morocco), and India.
♦ Fragrance: Deep, sweet, warming, longlasting, exhilarating, supremely exotic. Blends beautifully with rose, neroli, bergamot, petitgrain, sandalwood, citruses, palmarosa, geranium, rosewood.

There is no essential oil of jasmine: The oil is obtained by either enfleurage or solvent extraction (see Chapter 3). In enfleurage, fresh flowers are placed on top of a blend of fats (usually a mixture of pork fat, beef fat, and vegetable oils). The fat absorbs the fragrance released by the flower. The old flowers are removed every day and fresh flowers are placed on the fat. This process yields a product called pomade. The pomade is then washed with alcohol to remove the fats, and the alcohol is removed through vacuum distillation to produce the absolute from enfleurage.

Enfleurage is very time consuming and has generally been abandoned; only a few producers are still using this process. Currently, natural fats are replaced by a solvent (hexane, a petroleum derivative). The products obtained are called concrete (usually waxy) and absolute. Jasmine absolute is brown and rather viscous.

With rose and neroli, jasmine is one of the major "noble" oils of perfumery. It is also one of the most expensive oils; therefore it is very often adulterated. If rose is the oil of love, jasmine is certainly the oil of romance and was revered as such in the Hindu and Muslim traditions. It inspired burning lascivious songs by the Arab poets. In the harem, the prince's favorite soaked in a jasmine-scented bath and received an elaborate jasmine massage to induce sensual ecstasy in her lover.

Supremely sensual, jasmine is certainly the best aphrodisiac that aromatherapy can offer. It should not be considered a mere sexual stimulant, though. Jasmine releases inhibition, liberates imagination, and develops exhilarating playfulness. In a way, the power of jasmine can only be fully experienced by real lovers, as it has the power to transcend physical love and fully release both male and female sexual energy. It is the best stimulant of the sexual chakra and is recommended for any type of kundalini work.

Medicinal properties: Aphrodisiac, stimulant of sexual chakra; antidepressant; childbirth preparation.

Indications: Impotence, frigidity; anxiety, depression, lethargy, lack of confidence; postnatal depression; makes a fine perfume.

Labiatae: Plants of Heat

Essential oils of this family include basil, hyssop, lavender, lavandin (see lavender), marjoram, melissa, mints (pennyroyal, peppermint, spearmint) oregano, patchouli, rosemary, *Salvia* (clary sage, sage), spike (see lavender), thyme. While medicinal plants are the exception in most families, all Labiatae have some curative power, which indicates their special relationship to humans. This phenomenon is due to the extraordinary influence of the cosmic forces of heat on the formation of the family. This calorific nature leads to the formation of essential oils.

Labiatae have special predilection for open spaces; dry, rocky slopes; and sunny mountains, where their most characteristic species appear (lavender, rosemary, sage, thyme). They prefer median climatic regions: all around the Mediterranean and far from tropical and cold areas. Many Labiatae are culinary herbs, which indicates their affinity for the digestive processes. Their fragrance is invigorating, stimulating, fiery, reawakening. There are no bland, gloomy, ecstatic, or narcotic notes in this family.

Finally, many Labiatae (basil, peppermint, rosemary, thyme) have the power to develop chemotypes (see Chapter 4). This seems to indicate a strong potential for adaptability in the family, which could be interpreted as immunostimulant power. (Geranium is another plant with many chemotypes, and it is also considered an immunostimulant.)

Type of action: Warming, stimulating (vital center, metabolism); appeasing effect on overactive astral body; brings it back under the control of vital centers.

Domain of action: Organization of vital centers—metabolism, digestion, respiration, blood formation.

Indications: Weakness of vital centers (anemia, poor digestion, respiratory problems, diabetes); recommended for people with intense psychic activity (healers, mediums, etc.) to keep them from losing control and depleting their vitality.

Basil (Ocymum basilicum)

♦ Produced in India, Egypt, Comoro Islands, Reunion.
♦ Distillation of the herb: The oil is yellow.
♦ Fragrance: Pleasant, anisey, with a minty note.
♦ Used in perfumery for its top green note; blends well with bergamot or geranium.

There are several chemotypes of basil (there is even a cinnamon basil); the most commonly used is the methychavicol type (Reunion and Comoro Islands), as well as the eugenol type. One of the sacred plants of India, where it is dedicated to Vishnu, basil is extensively used in Ayurvedic medicine. Its actions on the digestive and nervous systems have been acknowledged in both Indian and occidental medicine.

Organs: Neurovegetative and digestive systems.

Medicinal properties: Nervous tonic, antispasmodic, cephalic; stomachic, intestinal antiseptic; stupefying at high doses.

Indications: Mental fatigue, migraine, insomnia, depression, mental strain; dyspepsia, gastric spasms; intestinal infections; facilitates birth and nursing.

Hyssop (Hyssopus officinalis)

♦ Produced in France, Spain, southern Europe.
♦ Distillation of the whole plant in flower: The oil is golden-yellow.

♦ Fragrance: nicely aromatic, reminiscent of sage, marjoram, and lavender.

One of the sacred plants of the Hebrews, hyssop *(esobh)* was prescribed by Hippocrates, Galen, and Dioscorides for its curative power on the respiratory system. The ancient pharmacopeia mention it as the major ingredient in numerous preparations, elixirs, and syrups.

Hyssop grows all over southern Europe and western Asia on dry, rocky slopes, but its finest varieties grow above three thousand feet in the sunny meadows of the southern Alps. Its abundant leaf system and its camphor-like scent indicate its special affinity for the respiratory system.

Organs: Lungs.

Medicinal properties: Expectorant (liquify bronchial secretions), antitussive, emollient; antispasmodic; tonic (especially heart and respiration); hypertensive agent, regulates blood pressure; digestive, stomachic; sudorific, febrifuge; cicatrizant, vulnerary.

Indications: Hypotension; respiratory diseases (asthma, bronchitis, catarrh, cough, tuberculosis); poor digestion, dyspepsia, flatulence; dermatitis, eczema, wounds; syphilis; urinary stones.

Lavender *(Lavandula officinalis)*

♦ One of the most precious essential oils.
♦ Produced in France, Spain, countries of the former Soviet Union
♦ Distillation of flowers: The oil is clear, yellowish-green.
♦ Fragrance: Clean, classic, appeasing.
♦ Best variety: "Lavender fine"; others: Mayette, materonne.

Lavender was a favorite aromatic used by the Romans in their baths (the word comes from the Latin *lavare*). Dioscorides, Pliny, and Galen mention it as a stimulant, tonic, stomachic, and carminative. It has always been used in perfumery and cosmetics and blends well with a great number of essential oils, adding a light floral note to almost any preparation.

Far from the ardor of rosemary, lavender emanates a noble, mellow peacefulness. Its blue flowers bloom at the top of a structure resembling a seven-branched candlestick; they give a clean, soothing scent that is one of our most beautiful perfumes.

The finest quality grows above three thousand feet on the sunny slopes of the southern Alps and up to the mountain top. Lavender likes air, space, light, and warmth. It has an appeasing action on the astral body; it tones and soothes the nervous system and is beneficial for the respiratory system.

Medicinal properties: Calming, analgesic, antispasmodic, anticonvulsive, antidepressant; antiseptic, healing; cytophylactic; diuretic, antirheumatic; insect repellent.

Indications: Respiratory diseases (asthma, bronchitis, catarrh, influenza, whooping cough, throat infections); sinusitis; migraine, depression, convulsions, nervous tension, fainting, insomnia, neurasthenia, palpitations; infectious diseases; skin diseases: abscess, acne dermatitis. eczema, pediculosis, psoriasis; burns, wounds; leukorrhea; cystitis, mucus discharge; insect bites.

Lavandin *(Lavandula fragrans, L. delphinensis)*

The lavandins are hybrids of true lavender and spike; their essential oils have a lower ester content and contain some camphor. Their fragrance is not as refined as that of lavender; their medicinal properties are similar, to a lesser degree.

Main varieties: Super and abrialis (the finest), grosso.

Veterinary uses: Antiseptic, vulnerary, dermatitis, scabies.

Spike *(Lavandula spica)*

Spike grows below two thousand feet. Its essential oils contain some camphor; it calms the ebrospinal activity. It is also used as an insecticide and for veterinary purposes.

Marjoram (Origanum marjorana, Marjorana hortensi)

+ Other variety: Wild spanish marjoram *(Thymus mastichina).*
+ Produced in Spain (wild Spanish marjoram), Egypt, North Africa, Hungary.
+ Distillation of the plant in flower.
+ Fragrance: Sweet, appeasing, one of the nicest of Labiatae oils.
+ Used in perfumery and cosmetics; blends well with lavender and bergamot.

Marjoram was grown in ancient Egypt, and Greeks and Romans used it to weave crowns for the newly married. According to mythology, Aphrodite, goddess of love and fecundity, picked marjoram on Mount Ida to heal the wounds of Enea. According to Dioscorides, it tones and warms the nerves; Pliny recommends it for poor digestion and a weak stomach; and Culpepper praises its warming and comforting effects.

Rather than altitude and rocks, marjoram prefers the light warm soil of gardens. The plant is sweet looking and delicate, with small, round, soft, velvety leaves and cute little white flowers, almost hidden among the leaves. Its gentle and appeasing fragrance has a warming and comforting effect, hence its beneficent action on the nervous system. Marjoram also has a warming action on the metabolism and genital organs.

Organs: Peripheral nervous system.

Medicinal properties: Antispasmodic, calming, sedative, analgesic, anaphrodisiac; hypotension, arterial vasodilator; digestive; narcotic in high doses.

Indications: Spasms (digestive, pulmonary), insomnia, migraine, nervous tension, neurasthenia, anxiety; hypertension; dyspepsia, flatulence; arthritis, rheumatic pain.

Melissa *(Melissa officinalis)*

+ Produced in France.
+ Distillation of the plant.
+ Fragrance: Fresh, lemony, very pleasant.

Melissa (sometimes called balm or lemon balm, or *citronelle* in French) has a very low yield (about 0.05 percent). The production of the oil had been virtually abandoned until the late 1980s when a few French producers started distilling it again. It is a very expensive oil and is therefore widely adulterated (most common additions are lemongrass, citronella, and *Litsea cubeba*). So-called melissa oil has been sold, especially in England, at a fraction of the production cost of true melissa oil. While total world production of melissa oil was less than fifty pounds in 1988, total sales worldwide could have been well over one thousand pounds (another miracle of modern technology)! Patricia Davis, in her excellent *Aromatherapy: An A–Z*, warns against possible skin irritations when using melissa oil externally. One wonders whether she used true melissa oil in the first place, since most of what is available for purchase is adulterated.

The plant is named after the Greek nymph Melissa, protectress of the bees. In spring, when several queens are born in the same beehive, the swarm splits into several smaller swarms, and each has to look for a new hive. Fresh leaves were traditionally crushed on empty hives to attract the migrant swarms.

Melissa is a gentle and humble-looking plant with pale green leaves and small white flowers. There emanates from the whole plant a natural kindness that is soothing and comforting in itself. Melissa was traditionally considered calming and uplifting; it is soothing, relieves tension, and is, with rose and neroli, one of the major oils of the heart chakra.

Melissa seems to thrive on iron. It likes the vicinity of houses, especially in the country where nails and other pieces of scrap iron are often buried around habitations. When I was a wildcrafter, the place where I could find the most abundant crop of melissa was an abandoned iron mine. This indicates a possible

antianemic and immunostimulant property; melissa has been known to strengthen vitality.

Medicinal properties: Antispasmodic, calming, sedative, soothing; antidepressant, uplifting; digestive; antivirus; stimulant of the heart chakra.

Indications: Insomnia; migraine, nervous tension, neurasthenia, anxiety; cold sores, shingles; emotional shock, grief.

Mints: Pennyroyal, Peppermint, Spearmint

Pluto once fell in love with the nymph Mintha, but his wife, the jealous Proserpine, changed her into the plant that is now named after her. According to Pliny, "The scent of mint awakens the mind and its taste excites the appetite and the stomach." Its fortifying and stimulating qualities have been acknowledge by Roman and Greek physicians.

There are about twenty species in the genus *Mentha*, growing all over the world. They like abundant light and deep, humid soils. In them, the warmth principle struggles against an adverse principle of cold and water, hence there is a warming, stimulating, curative power, good for resolving congestion cramps and swelling and to promote menstruation virility. On the other hand, mints also have vivifying, refreshing, and appeasing qualities.

Common medicinal properties of the genus Mentha: Stimulant of the nervous system, general tonic, antispasmodic; stomachic, digestive, carminative; hepatic, cholagogue; expectorant; emmenagogue;

febrifuge; antiseptic.

Indications: Gastralgia, dyspepsia, nausea, flatulence, vomiting; mental fatigue, migraine, headache, fainting, neuralgia; dysmenorrhea; hepatic disorders; cold, cough, asthma, bronchitis; neuralgia.

Pennyroyal *(Mentha pelugium)*

+ Produced in Spain, North Africa.
+ Distillation of the plant.
+ Fragrance: Resembles peppermint, but harsher.

Specific medicinal properties and indications: Amenorrhea *(warning: pennyroyal is abortive at high doses);* splenetic.

Peppermint *(Mentha piperita)*

+ Produced all over the world, the United States being the biggest producer; the finest quality comes from England and southern France.
+ Distillation of the plant.
+ Numerous uses in perfumery, cosmetics, and food industry (liquors, sauces, drinks, candies, etc.)

Mentha piperita has several subspecies and chemotypes *(Mentha piperita* var. *bergamia* or chemotype linalol, etc.), none of them being commercially distilled as far as I know.

Specific indications: Impotence.

Spearmint (Mentha viridis)

The fragrance of spearmint is very similar to that of peppermint, but is fresher and less harsh. Its therapeutic activity is approximately the same.

Oregano *(Origanum vulgare, O. compactum, Coridothymus capitatus)*

+ Produced in Spain, North Africa, Greece (many subspecies).
+ Distillation of the herb: The oil is brownish-red.
+ Fragrance: Burning, spicy, strongly aromatic.

Although the ancients often grouped different species under this name, oregano had been considered an essential aromatic plant for medicine and for cooking since antiquity. Theophrastes, Aristotle, and Hippocrates praised its beneficent action on respiratory diseases, ulcers, burns, and poor digestion.

A rustic variant of marjoram, oregano grows wild all over Europe and Asia; however, only the Mediterranean varieties yield a significant amount of essential oils. Their hot, almost burning quality indicates their beneficent action on infectious diseases, infected wounds, and inflammations.

Medicinal properties: Antiseptic, antitoxic, antivirus; antispasmodic, sedative; expectorant; analgesic, counterirritant.

Indications: Infectious diseases, disinfection; bronchopulmonary diseases; rheumatism; pediculosis; amenorrhea.

Patchouli *(Pogostemon patchouli)*

+ Produced in India, Malaysia, Burma, Paraguay.
+ The leaves are dried and fermented prior to distillation: The oil is thick, brown to greenish-brown.

- Fragrance: Strong, sweet, musty, very persistent.
- Used in dermatology, aesthetics, and skin care. One of the best fixatives, used in small amounts in oriental and rose perfumes.

Patchouli essential oil was part of the *materia medica* in Malaysia, China, India, and Japan, where it was used for its stimulant, tonic, stomachic, and febrifuge properties. It was a renowned antidote against insect and snake bites. The Indians also used it to scent their fabrics, especially the famous Indian shawls so fashionable in England in the nineteenth century. The oil contains patchoulene and other products close to azulene.

One of the most tropical Labiatae, patchouli is a plant of excessive warmth and water; however, its large leaves and its morphology indicate that these energies are not fully dominated. Therefore, although it is a stimulant and tonic at low doses, good for dissipating the type of lethargy related to such energies (sluggishness, inertia), it becomes sedative or even stupefying at high doses. Its antiinflammatory and decongestive properties also derive from these characteristics.

Because the oil is produced after a period of fermentation, it has certain control over all processes of stagnation, putrefaction, and aging (uses in skin care and rejuvenation). *Opus niger* (black work), which in the physical world is a process of fermentation and putrefaction, is one of the major phases of the alchemist's work, a phase conducive to the illumination of the adept after cold burn-

ing of all impurities and decantation. Patchouli is then a product of fermentation in the alchemical sense. It has powerful action on the psychic centers on a metaphysical level.

Medicinal properties: Decongestive, antiphlogistic, antiinflammatory, tissue regenerator, fungicide, antiinfectious, bactericide; stimulant (nervous system) at low doses; sedative at high doses; rejuvenating to the skin; insect repellent.

Indications: Mucus discharge, sluggishness; skin care (seborrhea, eczema, dermatitis, impetigo, herpes, cracked skin, wrinkles); anxiety, depression; insect and snake bites.

Rosemary (Rosamarinus officinalis)

- Produced all around the Mediterranean sea.
- Distillation of the herb: Oil almost colorless.
- Fragrance: Fiery, aromatic, invigorating, with a dominant note reminiscent of eucalyptus (for the Spanish and North African varieties) and of frankincense (more pronounced in the French and Yugoslavian varieties).

Like thyme, but to a lesser degree, rosemary has developed several chemotypes, growing in fairly distinct climatic areas. The phenol–cineol chemotype grows in North Africa (Morocco and Tunisia), the cineol chemotype grows in Spain, and the verbenon chemotype grows in southern France, Corsica, northern Italy, and Yugoslavia.

This vigorous, thick bush with a predilection for rocky, sunny slopes grows all around the Mediterranean, from the seashore to about two thousand feet. It has been used extensively since antiquity for medicine and in cooking, as well as for rituals. Highly praised in the Middle Ages and the Renaissance, it appeared in various formulas such as the famous "water of the Queen of Hungary," a rejuvenating liquor. At the age of seventy-two, when she was gouty and paralytic, Elizabeth of Hungary received the recipe from an angel (or a monk) and she recovered health and beauty. Madame de Sevigny recommended rosemary water for sadness.

A calorific plant above all, rosemary, according to Rudolf Steiner, fortifies the vital center and its action of other constituents of the human being. It restores the balance of the calorific body and activates the blood processes (blood is the privileged medium of the healing principle in the human body.) It is thus recommended for anemia, insufficient menstruation, and troubles of blood irrigation. Its acts on the liver as well.

A better irrigation of the organs eases the action of astral and viral forces and stimulates metabolism: rosemary is digestive and sudorific; it promotes the assimilation of sugar (in diabetes) and is indicated to rebuild the nervous system after long, intense intellectual activity.

Organs: Liver, gallbladder.

Medicinal properties: General stimulant, cariotonic, stimulant of adrenocortical glands; cholagogue, hepatobiliary stimulant (increase biliary secretion); pulmonary antiseptic; diuretic, sudorific; antirheumatismal, antineuralgic, rubefacient; healing of wounds and burns.

Indications: Hepatobiliary disorders (cholecystitis, cirrhosis, gallstone, hypercholesterolaemia, jaundice); general weakness, anemia, asthenia, debility, menstruation; mental fatigue, mental strain, loss of memory; colds, bronchitis, whooping cough; rheumatism, gout; hair loss, dandruff; skin care; wounds, burns; scabies, pediculosis.

Salvia

With over five hundred species, the genus *Salvia* is the most important of the Labiatae family. *Salvia officinalis* likes chalky rocks and the desert mountains of Spain, Greece, Dalmatia, and the Balkans. Its fragrance is severe, solemn, earthy, and harsh. Its well developed leaves and large odoriferous flowers shaped to receive the bodies of bees indicate its affinity for all processes of life and creation—even procreation. *S. sclarea* goes even further; reduced for years to a few small leaves close to the ground, it suddenly develops wide, thick leaves and extravagant flowers atop high, square stems, suggesting the quiet confidence and radiance of a pregnant woman. It was preeminently the plant of women in their creative process and was particularly indicated to induce and promote pregnancy.

Clary Sage (*Salvia sclarea*)

♦ Produced in southern France, countries of the former Soviet Union, United States.
♦ Distillation of the plant: The oil is clear.

♦ Fragrance: Pleasant, sweet with floral notes, slightly musky.
♦ Widely used as a fixative in cosmetics and perfumery.

Clary sage is preferred to other sages for long cures (with no toxicity).

Organs: Female genitals.

Medicinal properties and indications: Similar to those of *S. officinalis*, with a special emphasis on women's complaints pertaining to menstruation, leukorrhea, and frigidity.

Sage (*Salvia officinalis*)

♦ Produced in Spain, Yugoslavia, France.
♦ Distillation of leaves and flowers.
♦ Fragrance: Harsh, aromatic (*S. lavandulifolia*, growing in northern Spain, is finer and milder).

Renowned since antiquity, the "salvia salvatrix" of the Romans is one of the most powerful and versatile medicinal plants. Indeed, *Cur moriatur homo, cui salvia crescit in horto?* (Why should he die, the one who grows sage in his garden?) That panacea, which preserves health and youth, was always recommended for conception and pregnancy.

The essential oil of sage is tonic at high doses and should not be taken internally for very long. It is not recommended for people with epileptic tendencies.

Organs: Liver, gallbladder, kidneys.

Medicinal properties: Tonic, stimulant (adrenocortical glands, nerves); antisudorific; antiseptic; diuretic; emmenagogue; hypertensive agent; aperitive, stomachic; depurative; astringent, vulnerary.

Indications: General weakness, anemia, asthenia, neurasthenia; hypotension; sterility, menopause, regulation of menstruation, birth preparation; perspiration, fever; hepatobiliary and kidney dysfunctions; nervous afflictions; bronchitis, asthma; mouth ulcers, stomatitis, tonsillitis, dermatitis; hair loss; wounds, ulcers.

Thyme (*Thymus vulgaris*)

♦ Produced in Morocco, Spain, France, Greece.
♦ The oil is obtained from branches and flowers. It is red or brownish-red liquid for the thymol-carvacrol chemotypes and clear to yellowish for the other chemotypes.
♦ Fragrance: Hot, spicy, aromatic for the thymol-carvacrol chemotypes, sweet to fresh and green for the others (citrusy for the citral chemotype, rose-like for the geraniol, etc.).

The genus *Thymus* produces many species, subspecies, and chemotypes all around the Mediterranean sea (see Appendix I). For some yet unknown reason, the same subspecies produces oils with totally different chemical compositions (this phenomenon, discovered only recently, is called chemotyping). It has been suggested that such variations may be caused by climatic and other environmental conditions. Thus, the burning hot thymol and carvacrol chemotypes would grow at lower altitudes and in dryer climates, while the milder geraniol, linalol, citral, and thuyanol chemotypes would grow at higher altitudes and milder climates. It has even been suggested that a plant of thyme transplanted from one climatic area to another begins to develop the characteristics of its new location (i.e., thyme growing in dryness at sea level would be thymol–carvacrol chemotype, but would become linalol or geraniol when transplanted to a high altitude).

As seductive as this theory might be, the reality is slightly different. There is, in the wild, a predominance of the thymol and carvacrol chemotypes in the dryer and warmer areas, while the milder chemotypes are more abundant under milder conditions. But more than seven years of wild harvesting of thyme have shown me that the different chemotypes can be found everywhere. Furthermore, most of the commercial production of chemotyped thyme comes from the same area of southern France, and several farmers grow all the chemotypes on their farms.

This tiny bush, with no special requirements for soil quality or the amount of humidity, is quite avid of warmth and light. It is helpful whenever inner warmth is poor or missing: excess of water, chilling tendencies, cold, and weakness of the vital center, especially when it is manifested at the level of lungs or stomach.

Thyme has been widely used for therapy since antiquity for its warming, stimulant, and cleansing properties. Thyme is able to create, by itself, almost the entire spectrum of fragrances demonstrated by the medicinal family: the Labiatae, from the hot burning thymol-carvacrol (reminiscent of oregano or savory) to the citral types similar to melissa,

through the linalol types (marjoram, lavender). This shows the amazing adaptability of the genus, its broad-spectrum curative power, and its incredible vital energy. Thymes certainly are among the major oils of aromatherapy.

Medicinal properties: General stimulant (physic, psychic, capillary circulation); antiseptic (lungs, intestine, genitourinary system); rubefacient; healing; balsamic, expectorant.

Indications: Asthenia, anemia, neurasthenia, nervous deficiency; infectious diseases (intestinal and urinary); pulmonary diseases (bronchitis, tuberculosis, asthma); poor digestion, fermentation; rheumatism, arthritis, gout; flu, influenza, sore throat; wounds.

Myrtaceae: Harmony and Equilibrium in the Interaction of the Four Elements, Fire, Air, Water, Earth

Essential oils of this family include cajeput, clove, eucalyptus, myrtle, niaouli, nutmeg, and tea tree. Other oils of interest are bay and red pepper. Myrtaceae grow in the tropical zones of every continent. Confronted with the powerful forces of earth and water in relation to strong tropical influences, Myrtaceae oppose a very structured formatting principle. The plants and trees of the family have a noble and harmonious aspect, which expresses the perfect equilibrium among the four elements in the constitution of the type. The astral sphere is never violent to etheric formatting forces: the type does not produce any poisonous plant.

The evergreen leaves are strong and simple. They open themselves to the supra vegetal and animal sphere in an intense floral process (pollination is accomplished by insects and birds). The sugar process is very strong in this family, which produces some delicious fruits: pomegranate, gooseberry, guava, myrtoloela fruits, and jabotica plums.

The deep penetration of tropical warmth into the leaf, the flower, the bark, and the wood generates etheric oils and aromatic resins. The family also produces some condiments (cloves, red pepper). Finally, they produce very hard woods, which reveals the healthy relation to this family with the earth element.

Type of action: Reequilibrating.

Domain of action: Metabolism, energy centers, lungs.

Indications: Respiratory diseases; metabolic or energetic lack of balance.

Cajeput (Melaleuca leucadendron)

♦ Produced in Malaysia and Far Eastern countries.
♦ Distillation of the leaves. The oil is yellowish-green.
♦ Fragrance: Penetrating, camphorlike.
♦ Used in numerous pectoral preparations, also used as insecticide and parasiticide.

In Malaysia and Java, cajeput oil was a traditional remedy for cholera and rheumatism.

Medicinal properties: General antiseptic (pulmonary, urinary, intestinal); antispasmodic, antineuralgic; sudorific; febrifuge.

Indications: Pulmonary diseases (bronchitis, tuberculosis); cystitis, urethritis; dysentery, diarrhea, amebiasis; rheumatism, rheumatic pains; earaches.

Clove (Eugenia caryophyllata)

♦ Produced in Molucca Islands, Madagascar, Zanzibar, Indonesia.
♦ Distillation of the dried buds. The oil is brown to dark brown.
♦ Clove stems and clove leaves are also distilled; they are of lower quality (especially the former) and are often used to adulterate clove bud oil.
♦ Fragrance: Hot, spicy, characteristic.
♦ Used in dentistry, pharmacy, food industry, perfumery.

Native of the Molucca Islands, clove is one of the best-known spices of the world, along with black pepper, cinnamon, and nutmeg. It was so precious in ancient times that it caused a few wars: its trade was almost exclusively controlled by the Portuguese, who possessed the Molucca Islands until the seventeenth century, when the Dutch drove them out. To better control the monopoly and raise prices, the Dutch destroyed all plantations except the one on Amboine Island. The French finally stole a few plants to start new plantations in Guyana, Zanzibar, Reunion, and Trinidad. Clove oil was long used in dentistry as an analgesic.

In the clove tree, the terrestrial forces of the roots rise into the floral area: the essential oil of the buds, heavier than water and not easily volatile, is heavy and burning, which reveals that the fire cosmic forces have been strongly drawn into the ground. This special interaction of the fire and earth energies in the floral area results in a strong action on the metabolism: clove stimulates the digestion of heavy food and regulates the digestive tract.

Medicinal properties: Antineuralgic, analgesic; powerful antiseptic, cicatrizant; stomachic, carminative; aphrodisiac, stimulant; parasiticide.

Indications: Toothache; prevention of infectious diseases; physical and intellectual asthenia (to strengthen memory); dyspepsia, gastric fermentation, flatulence; impotence; infected wounds, ulcers.

Eucalyptus (Eucalyptus globulus)

♦ Produced in Australia, Spain, Portugal.
♦ Distillation of the leaves: The oil is yellow to red.
♦ Fragrance: Fresh, balsamic, camphorlike.
♦ Numerous uses in pharmacy.

Native of Australia, where it was regarded as a general cure-all by the Aborigines and later by the white settlers, eucalyptus has now spread almost entirely over the tropical and subtropical parts of the world. It has a long tradition of use in medicine, and its essential oil is one of the most powerful and versatile remedies.

Eucalyptus is one of the tallest trees in the world and is deeply rooted: its roots go amazingly deep in the ground to find aquifer veins and strongly draw water to its vigorous branches and leaves. It is used to drain marshy areas and cleanse them from mosquitos. It grows incredibly fast,

but forms nevertheless a very strong wood, fairly resistant to rot. The leaves, shaped like swords, are oriented in such a way as to avoid a strong exposure to the sun, and allow the light to go through the whole tree and reach the ground. Eucalyptus energetically draws the solidifying forces of earth and water into the clear and dry area of air and light, where it attracts astral force for the production of essential oils—hence its action on the urinary and pulmonary systems. It is especially beneficent in the treatment of pulmonary inflammation and excessive mucosity.

Medicinal properties: General antiseptic (especially pulmonary and urinary); balsamic, expectorant, antispasmodic; hypoglycemic; febrifuge; stimulant; cicatrizant, vulnerary; parasiticide.

Indications: Respiratory diseases (asthma, bronchitis, tuberculosis, flu, sinusitis); urinary infections; diabetes; fevers; rheumatism; intestinal parasites (ascaris, oxyurids).

Myrtle (Myrtus communis)

♦ Produced in North Africa.
♦ Distillation of branches: The oil is yellow.
♦ Fragrance: Fresh, close to eucalyptus.

The Greeks and Romans used myrtle for pulmonary and urinary diseases. In the sixteenth century, the leaves and flowers were used for skin care; they served in the preparation of "angel water," a renowned tonic and astringent lotion. The medicinal properties of myrtle closely resemble those of eucalyptus.

Specific therapeutic indications: Skin care.

Niaouli (Melaleuca viridiflora)

♦ Produced in Madagascar, Australia, and New Caledonia.
♦ Distillation of the leaves: The oil (also called "gomenol") is yellow.
♦ Fragrance: Strong, camphorlike, balsamic, close to eucalyptus.
♦ Same medicinal properties and indications as eucalyptus.

Specific therapeutic indications: Stimulating to tissues (promotes local circulation and leukocyte and antibody activity); infected wounds, ulcers, burns.

Nutmeg (Myristica fragrans, Myristicaceae)

♦ Produced in the West Indies, Indonesia, Java.
♦ Distillation of the nuts: The oil is colorless.
♦ The nut is surrounded by a fleshy shell, which, by distillation, yields an essential oil called mace oil; it is of lower quality than nutmeg oil, with similar composition and properties.
♦ Fragrance: Spicy, peppery, aromatic.
♦ Some applications in pharmaceutical preparations; few uses in perfumery; widely used for the manufacture of spirits and elixirs.

First mentioned in the fifth century, nutmeg was introduced to the Occident by Arabian merchants. Portugal had the monopoly of its trade until 1605, when the Dutch took over their possessions. The plantations were placed under military protection, and prices were kept high by systematic destruction of the trees growing in nearby islands. Huge amounts of the spice were even burned at intervals to keep the price high. Pierre Poivre finally stole a few plants in 1768, and the nutmeg tree was then grown in other tropical countries.

Nutmeg has been highly appreciated since the early middle ages and was an ingredient of numerous balms, elixirs, and unguents. In 1704 Pollini wrote more than eight hundred pages on the invaluable virtues of nutmeg. He concluded that "in good health or disabled, alive or dead, nobody can do without this nut, the most salutary medicine!" It is indeed a very powerful tonic and stimulant.

Organs: Digestive system.

Medicinal properties: Tonic, stimulant (nervous system, circulation); digestive, intestinal antiseptic; sedative, analgesic; aphrodisiac; stupefying and toxic at high doses (delirium, hallucinations, fainting).

Indications: Digestive problems, intestinal infections, flatulence; asthenia; nervous and intellectual fatigue; impotence; rheumatic pain, neuralgia.

Tea Tree (Melaleuca alternifolia)

♦ Produced in Australia.
♦ Distillation of the leaves: The oil is yellowish.
♦ Fragrance: Strong, camphorlike, balsamic, pungent.

A relative newcomer to the aromatherapy scene, tea tree has quickly become a universal panacea, first-aid kit, or cure-all. It is (with oregano and savory) one of the oils whose medical and antiseptic properties are the most widely documented. Research in Australia begun in the late 1920s showed the amazing anti-infectious power of the oil. During World War II, it was even included in military first-aid kits in tropical areas. Extensive research during the 1970s and 1980s (Morton Walker, Dr. Eduardo F. Pena, Dr. Paul Belaiche) has showed its strong antifungus action. Its wide range of action and its low toxicity make it an ideal home remedy for inclusion in any aromatherapy first-aid kit (with lavender and eucalyptus).

A somewhat small tree with needle-type leaves (similar to cypress), tea tree shows an amazing vitality. Before becoming a rare commodity when the demand for its oil increased dramatically in the 1980s, tea tree was considered a weed—a real plague, in fact—and farmers could not get rid of it. Cut down to the roots, it grows flourishing, thick foliage in less than two years. Even more than eucalyptus, it likes swampy, marshy areas. Unlike eucalyptus, though, its leaves are hardly developed, which indicates a predominance of earth, fire, and water over air. Tea tree yields one of the best antifungus, anti-infectious, and antiseptic oils, but eucalyptus works better on respiratory conditions. Finally, the amazing vitality of tea tree indicates its strong immunostimulant properties.

Medicinal properties: Antifungus (*Candida albicans, Trichomonas*); anti-infectious; general antiseptic (especially urinary); immunostimulant; balsamic, expectorant; cicatrizant, vulnerary; parasiticide.

Indications: Fungal infections (ringworm, athlete's foot, vaginitis, thrush, *Candida albicans*); urinary infections, cystitis; infected wounds, ulcers, sores, and any infectious condition; cold sores, blisters, chickenpox; acne; rashes, anal and genital pruritis, genital herpes; intestinal parasites; surgery preparation (prevention); low immune system; dandruff, hair care.

Pepper (*Piper nigrum*, Piperaceae)

- Produced in India, Java, Sumatra, China.
- Distillation of the seeds. The oil is yellow-green.
- Fragrance: Characteristic.
- Few uses in perfumery and food industry.

One of the most ancient spices, pepper was mentioned in Chinese and Sanskrit texts a few thousand years ago. In the Western countries, it was the most valued spice and was used as currency in the Middle Ages. The essential oil of pepper was described by Valerius Cordius in his *Compendium Aromatorium* in 1488. It is traditionally indicated as a stimulant and tonic and whenever there is an excess of cold or water.

Medicinal properties: Stimulant, tonic (especially digestive and nervous systems); digestive, stomachic, antitoxic; heating, drying, comforting; analgesic, rubefacient; aphrodisiac; stimulant of the root chakra.

Indications: Digestive problems (dyspepsia, flatulence, loss of appetite, food poisoning); fever, cold, catarrh, cough, influenza; neuralgia, toothache, rheumatic aches; muscular pain, sport massage (preparation for effort); gonorrhea; impotence; ungroundedness.

Rose (*Rose centifolia* and *R. damascena*, Rosaceae)

- Produced in Bulgaria, Morocco, Turkey.
- The rose buds are picked during a few morning hours only, right after the dew, and distilled immediately: The oil is rather thick, yellow to greenish-yellow.
- Fragrance: Characteristic.

One of the most expensive essential oils, rose oil is almost always adulterated with substances like geranium, lemongrass, palmarosa, and terpene alcohols (geraniol, citronellol, rhodinol, linalol, nerol, etc.). The processes of adulteration have become so refined that is almost impossible to disclose frauds. Real rose oil is used only in very high-grade perfumes. Rose water is widely used in cosmetics and perfumery.

Whether it sprang from the blood of Venus, the blood of Adonis, or the sweat of Mohammed, the rose—the queen of flowers—is certainly immemorial. Praised by the poets, revered in the sacred books, and offered to the kings and the gods, the rose is a traditional symbol of love. Bunches of roses were found in the sarcophagus of Tutankhamon, offered by the Queen Ankhsenamon as a token of her love. When the Persian Emperor Djihanguyr married the Princess Nour-Djihan, a canal encircling the gardens was filled with rose water.

Droplets of oil were noticed floating on the top of the water; that was the beginning of the production of the famous Persian rose oil.

Rose water is an excellent skin tonic, recommended for any type of skin; it is good for wrinkles, inflammation, redness, and sensitive skin and is indicated for ophthalmia.

Organs and functions: Female reproductive system, heart chakra.

Medicinal properties: Uplifting, antidepressant, tonic; astringent, hemostatic; depurative; aphrodisiac; stimulant of the heart chakra.

Indications: Nervous tension, depression, insomnia, headache; skin care (wrinkles, eczema, sensitive skin, aged skin); disorders of the female reproductive system (frigidity, sterility, uterine disorders); hemorrhage; impotence; emotional shock, grief, depression.

Rosewood (*Aniba roseaodora*, Lauraceae)

- Produced in Brazil.
- Distillation of the chopped wood: The oil is clear to pale yellow.
- Fragrance: Very sweet, floral, woody. Blends very well with almost any oil.

Rosewood oil is one of the major oils of perfumery, where it is used as a middle note. It was little used in aromatherapy until recently. Although it does not have any dramatic curative power (like tea tree or lavender), I find it very useful, especially for skin care. It is mild and safe to use. It is also very useful in blending and helps to give body to a blend and to round sharp edges. Rosewood is excellent for any type of body care or skin care preparation (bath oils, lotions, masks, facials).

Medicinal properties: Cellular stimulant, tissue regenerator; uplifting, antidepressant, tonic; calming, cephalic.

Indications: Headache nausea; skin care (sensitive skin, aged skin, wrinkles, general skin care); scars, wounds.

Rutaceae: Processes of Subdued Topical Heat

Essential oils of this family include bergamot, grapefruit, lemon, lime, neroli, orange, petitgrain, tangerine. Other oils of interest are rue *(Ruta graveolens). Warning: this oil is highly toxic and should be used with great care.*

Most Rutaceae grow in the tropical area; in these areas, they are mostly small thorny trees with hard wood, which is often resinous, and firm green leaves. Their beautiful abundant flowers shaped like symmetrical stars exhale a delicious, sweet, slightly exhilarating fragrance. The scent of the leaves is fresh and comforting with a hint of bitterness. The trees develop juicy acid fruits (citrus) or small, hot, spicy berries.

The general therapeutic activity of Rutaceae concerns the interaction of warmth and fluid in the body. The oils reduce proliferations, distensions, inflammations, and looseness; they strengthen the astral body, and their formatting forces are activated by air and warmth.

Members of the genus *Citrus* are listed and discussed here. Neroli essential oil is obtained by distillation of the flowers.

Distillation of the leaves gives petitgrain. The essential oils of bergamot, grapefruit, lemon, lime, orange, and tangerine are extracted from the peel of the fruits by cold pressure.

Extremely prolific (each tree can produce up to one hundred fruits), deeply rooted, and densely ramified, citruses perfectly control the interaction of the two powerful opposite flows of forces: centrifugal forces that strongly draw up the terrestrial forces, charging them with vitalized fluid elements of a tropical luxuriance, and cosmic forces of light and warmth that are absorbed by the leaves, the bark, the wood, and the fruit. Their energetic floral process and their light, suave, almost ethereal and very pervasive fragrance suggest an etheric organism intensely penetrated by the peripheral astral sphere. Citrus fruits are liquid like a berry, but are surrounded with a tough envelope shaped by the forces of air and warmth.

Citruses strive against the dissolving centrifugal forces of the tropical world. Their action is refreshing, vivifying, and tonic and tends to gather the constitutive elements of the body.

The floral area expresses a soft, delicious, appeasing exhilaration, indicative of the remarkable sedative, antidepressant power of the blossoms. The fragrance of the thick, vigorous leaves is less refined, more hearty and grounded, and slightly bitter. Their action is then invigorating, comforting, and almost materialistic, even compared with the ethereal neroli.

Type of action: Cooling, refreshing;

sedative (flowers); control of liquid processes, secretion (fruits).

Domain of action: Digestive system, kidneys, liver; nervous system.

Indications: Inflammations, infectious diseases; excess of liquids (obesity); oversensitivity, nervous tension.

Bergamot (Citrus bergamia)

- Produced in Italy, the Ivory Coast, and Guinea.
- Cold pressure of the rind of the fruit: The oil is yellowish-green, emerald.
- Fragrance: Sweet, citrusy, with a floral note.
- Widely used in perfumery; blends perfectly with almost any oil; and makes a perfect top note.

Medicinal properties: Antispasmodic; antiseptic; cordial, tonic, stomachic, digestive; vulnerary.

Indications: Colic, intestinal infection, intestinal parasites, stomatitis; skin care.

Grapefruit (Citrus paradisi)

- Mostly produced in the United States.
- Various uses in perfumery and food industry.
- Blends fairly well with other citrus oils, geranium, cedarwood.

Specific therapeutic indications: Obesity.

Lemon (Citrus limonum)

- Produced all around the Mediterranean and in California, Brazil, and Argentina.
- Extraction by cold pressure of the skin:

The oil is yellow to yellowish-green.
- Numerous uses in perfumery, cosmetics, pharmacy, and the food and soap industries.
- Blends well with many oils; makes a nice green note.
- One of the most versatile essential oils in aromatherapy.

Profusely thorny, with very thick leaves and the most acid fruit of the vegetable kingdom, the small lemon tree gives an impression of fresh, optimistic, fearless strength. Here the fire/water dialectic is resolved on the cooling side. The fruit is tightly structured under a fairly tough skin; expansion, dilation, and inflation are under control.

Medicinal properties: Bactericide, antiseptic, stimulant of leukocytosis; stimulant, tonic; stomachic, carminative; diuretic; hepatic; liquefy the blood, hypotensive agent; depurative; antirheumatic.

Indications: Infectious diseases; anemia, asthenia; varicosis, arteriosclerosis, hyperviscosity of the blood, hypertension; rheumatism; dyspepsia, flatulence; hepatic congestion; skin diseases, skin care; herpes.

Lime (Citrus limetta)

- Produced in Florida, Central America, Caribbean Islands.
- The oil is extracted from the skin by cold pressure or distillation. The cold-pressed oil is far superior to the distilled oil; it is gold to yellowish-green.
- Fragrance: Fresh, green, very pleasant; similar to bergamot for the cold-pressed oil; much heavier for the distilled oil.

The indications and various uses of lime are similar to those of lemon (although its refreshing quality is more pronounced). It makes a very good aftershave lotion.

Neroli (Orange Blossom, Citrus vulgaris)

♦ Produced in France, Spain, North Africa, Italy, and, recently, the Comoro Islands.
♦ One of the most expensive oils, therefore widely adulterated.
♦ Fragrance: One of the finest floral essences, sweet, suave, delicious, slightly euphoric.
♦ Used in expensive cologne and perfumes, it blends well with almost any oil and is useful as the heart of a floral blend.

Real neroli (also called neroli biguarade) is extracted from bitter orange blossom (or *biguarade*). However, other citrus blossoms are sometimes distilled (sweet orange, lemon, mandarin). A native of China, where its flowers were traditionally used in cosmetics, orange trees now grow all around the Mediterranean, in the United States, and in Central and South America. Neroli was already being produced in the beginning of the sixteenth century. It became a fashionable perfume when the Duchess of Nerole started using it to scent her gloves.

The hydrolate obtained by distillation is more commonly known as orange-flower water; it is widely used for skin care and pastry-making. It is soothing, digestive, and carminative.

Medicinal properties: Antidepressant, antispasmodic, sedative; diminishes the amplitude of heart muscle contractions; aphrodisiac; stimulant of the heart chakra.

Indications: Insomnia, hysteria, anxiety, depression, nervous tension; palpitations; diarrhea related to stress; skin care (dry or sensitive skin); grief, emotional shock; mild remedy for infants' colics and to send them to sleep.

Orange (Citrus auranthium)

♦ Produced in Spain, North Africa, the United States, and Central and South America.
♦ The oil is orange.
♦ Numerous uses in perfumery and food industry.

Biguarade, or bitter orange, is even more thorny than lemon; the strong bitterness of its fruit indicates a special affinity for the liver. With sweet orange, qualities are softened: no more thorns, and the fruit is not totally edible. The water processes are less tight, and the soothing properties are more pronounced.

Medicinal properties: Febrifuge; stomachic, digestive; antispasmodic, sedative, cardiotonic.

Indications: Fever; indigestion, dyspepsia, flatulence, gastric spasms; skin care, wrinkles, dermatitis; nervous troubles.

Petitgrain (Bitter Orange Leaves)

♦ Areas of production: Same as neroli.
♦ Fragrance: Fresh, invigorating, slightly floral with a bitter note.

♦ Widely used in pharmacy and perfumery (the basic ingredient of good colognes). Blends well with almost any oil.

Like neroli, real petitgrain (or petitgrain biguarade) is obtained by distilling the leaves of the bitter orange tree. Petitgrain bergamot, petitgrain lemon, and petitgrain mandarin are also produced.

Specific therapeutic indications: Painful digestion, sedative of nervous system; tonic, intellectual stimulant, strengthens memory.

Tangerine (Citrus reticulata)

♦ Produced in Italy (mandarin) and the United States (tangerine).
♦ Mandarin oil is much finer than tangerine oil (a hybrid).
♦ Fragrance: Sweeter than orange, reminiscent of bergamot.

Native China, tangerine is the most delicate fruit; it was traditionally offered to the mandarins (hence the name mandarin). The medicinal properties of tangerine are very close to those of orange. The sedative and antispasmodic properties, however, are more pronounced.

Mandarin is certainly the softest of all citrus trees. The leaves are delicate, the fruit is very sweet, and the taste is quite refined. The peel is soft and the fragrance is almost exotic. The soothing action on the nervous centers is then quite pronounced.

Specific therapeutic indications: Calming, antispasmodic, hypnotic nervous tension, insomnia, epilepsy.

Sandalwood (Santalum album, Santalaceae)

♦ Produced in India, Indonesia, and China.
♦ Distillation of the inner wood: The oil is thick and yellow.
♦ Fragrance: Characteristic (persistent, woody, sweet, spicy, oriental).
♦ Very good fixative, widely used in high-class perfumes. Often adulterated.

A sacred tree of India, sandalwood is mentioned in the old Sanskrit and Chinese books. It is widely used as incense, in religious ceremonies, and in medicine and cosmetics.

Organs: Genitourinary tract.

Medicinal properties: Genitourinary antiseptic, diuretic; antidepressant, tonic, aphrodisiac; antispasmodic; astringent.

Indications: Genitourinary infections—gonorrhea, blennorrhoea, cystitis, colibacillosis; impotence.

Umbelliferae: Plants of the Air Element

Essential oils of this family include angelica, aniseed, caraway, carrot, coriander, cumin, fennel, and lovage. Other oils of interest are ammi-visnaga, aneth, asafetida, celery, galbanum, and parsley.

This family is characterized by the extreme division of the leaves, ending up in an aerial explosion in such plants as fennel or anise. The leaf is the origin of interaction and confrontation between air and water, light and darkness.

Umbelliferae obviously are very sensitive to this confrontation. The interaction of air, light, water, and earth through these extremely ramified leaves gives birth, in a contraction process, to a strong root or vigorous rhizome, which stays underground for one year or more. This subterranean organ draws the cosmic forces into the ground. Then vegetation grows rapidly in a radiating explosion, until it reaches the final bouquet of the inflorescence, with its radiating umbel—each branch of the umbel splitting again in umbellules.

The special interaction of this family with the air element is further emphasized by their ability to incorporate air within themselves in hollow stems, hollow seeds, and even hollow rhizomes.

In the archetypal plant, the interaction between the plant's etheric organism and the surrounding astral forces takes place in the flower area. This process is manifested in the colors and fragrance of the flower and the formation of nectar. Umbelliferae attract cosmic forces in the leaves, the stem, and even the rhizome. Their aromatic substances are therefore heavier, harsher, and less refined than floral scents.

Umbelliferae, in fact, start their fructification process in the leaves, or even the root. They produce some of the most tasty vegetables (carrot, celery, fennel) and condiments (parsley, coriander, chervil, anise, cumin, carvi, etc.).

In addition to this descending movement there is also an ascending movement of mucilages and gums, another characteristic of the family. The therapeutic action of Umbelliferae is then easy to understand. First, they have an affinity for the digestive system (especially the intestine) and a strong effect on the secretions and the glandular system. Finally, they are useful in respiratory diseases.

According to Robert Tisserand in *Aromatherapy to Heal and Tend the Body*, "Tissue regeneration in the livers of rats has been demonstrated in the essential oils, in particular the four seed oils—cumin, fennel, celery and parsley" (which all belong to the Umbelliferae family). Carrot seed oil has been used successfully to fight against the aging skin process.

Type of action: Accumulation/excretion, elimination; secretion (diuretic, sudorific, expectorant); regulation of the aerial processes in the organism (carminative, antispasmodic); tissue regeneration.

Domain of action: Digestive system (especially intestines), glandular system; respiratory system.

Indications: Digestive and intestinal problems, accumulation of gas; spasms (digestive, respiratory, circulatory); glandular problems.

Angelica (Angelica archangelica)

♦ Produced in Belgium, France, Poland.
♦ The oil is obtained from seeds or roots; it is almost colorless.
♦ Fragrance: Balsamic, nicely aromatic, slightly musky.

Several varieties of angelica grow in northern Europe, mainly *Angelica sylvestris* (wild) and *Angelica arch-*

angelica (domestic, cultured). The plant was highly valued by physicians of the Renaissance. Paracelsus reported that it was of great help during the epidemic of pestilence in Milan in 1510.

This vigorous prolific plant of the air element (with a hollow stem) grows in deep humid soils and rather cool temperate climates. (It grows wild by streams and irrigation canals.) Therefore, it is a typical plant of elimination. It helps to eliminate toxins, purify the bloody and lymph, and stimulate the glandular system. It is recommended for weakness and nervousness and for convalescents and old people.

Medicinal properties: Depurative, sudorific; stomachic, digestive, aperitive; stimulant, tonic, cephalic, revitalizing.

Indications: Nervous afflictions related to the digestive system (cramps, spasms, aerophagia, digestive migraine); weakness of stomach; asthenia, anemia, anorexia, rachitis, neurovegetative cardiopathies; lung diseases (bronchitis, flu, pneumonia, pleuresy); gout (compresses, massage).

Aniseed (Pimpinella anisum)

♦ Produced in Spain, Egypt, North Africa, countries of the former Soviet Union.
♦ Distillation of the seeds: The oil is slightly yellow.

Mentioned in the Vedas and the Bible, anise was considered one of the main medicinal plants in China, India, Egypt, Greece, and Rome. According to Pythagorus, it is an excellent carminative and appetizer.

Unlike most Umbelliferae, anise grows flowers and seeds in its first year. Only in a very dry climate can the seeds fully ripen. The forces of warmth are thus condensed in these small aniseeds, the taste of which is aqueous and fiery. The medicinal properties of anise are then the same as those of most plants of the type, but its antispasmodic expectorant power is accentuated, with a narcotic or even stupefying effect.

Medicinal properties: Stomachic, carminative, antispasmodic; general stimulant (digestive, respiratory, cardiac); galactogogue; diuretic; aphrodisiac; stupefying at high doses.

Indications: Nervous dyspepsia, aerophagia, gas accumulation, digestive migraines; insufficient milk (nursing mothers); impotence, frigidity; epilepsy.

Caraway (Carum carvi)

♦ Produced in northern Europe.
♦ Distillation of seeds: Oil is yellowish.

Caraway seed is used in pastries and delicatessen foods in northern Europe and the Arab countries. Its medicinal properties are very similar to those of aniseed.

Medicinal properties: Carminative; antispasmodic; general stimulant (digestive, respiratory, cardiac); diuretic.

Indications: Digestive and intestinal troubles; aerophagia, gas accumulation, fermentations; nervous dyspepsia, digestive migraine; scabies, mange (dogs) (see Valnet).

Carrot (Daucus carota)

♦ Produced in France, Egypt, India.
♦ Distillation of the seeds: The oil is slightly yellow.
♦ Fragrance: Characteristic (carrotlike).

Carrot has been used since the sixteenth century as a carminative, diuretic, and hepatic and for skin diseases.

Medicinal properties: Depurative, hepatic; emmenagogue; diuretic.

Indications: Jaundice, hepatobiliary disorders; favors menstruation and conception; skin diseases.

Coriander (Coriandrum sativum)

♦ Produced in North Africa, Spain, countries of the former Soviet Union.
♦ Distillation of the seeds: The oil is slightly yellow.
♦ Fragrance: Anise-y, musky, aromatic.

Seeds of coriander found in Egyptian sepulchers prove that it was already used by the time of Ramses II. Theophrasta, Hippocrates, Galen, and Pliny talk about its properties as a stimulant, carminative, and digestive.

Medicinal properties and indications: Same as all Umbelliferae (aerophagia, digestion, flatulence, spasms); stupefying at high doses.

Cumin (Cuminum cyminum)

♦ Produced in North Africa and the Far East.
♦ Distillation of the seeds: The oil is slightly yellow.
♦ Fragrance: Bitter, anise-y, aromatic.

Native of Egypt, cumin is a close relative of coriander. It was a traditional spice in the Middle East and is one of the ingredients of curry. It is an excellent digestive stimulant, which should, however, be used with great care, as it can provoke skin irritation.

Medicinal properties and indications: Same as all Umbelliferae (aerophagia, digestion, flatulence, spasms).

Fennel (Foeniculum vulgare)

♦ Produced in Spain, North Africa, India, Japan.
♦ Distillation of the seeds: The oil is yellowish.
♦ Fragrance: Strong, anisey, camphoric.
♦ Used in India, Egypt, China. In the Middle Ages, people used it to prevent witchcraft and as a protection against evil spirits.

Medicinal properties: Aperitive, stomachic, carminative; emmenagogue, galactogogue; diuretic; antispasmodic; laxative.

Indications: Dyspepsia, flatulence, digestive problems, aerophagia; amenorrhea, menopausal problems; insufficient milk; oliguria, obesity, kidney stones.

Lovage (Levisticum officinalis)

♦ Produced in France and Belgium.
♦ Distillation of the roots: The oil is slightly yellow.
♦ Fragrance: Musky, earthy.

Medicinal properties: Intestinal and kidney stimulant; diuretic; drainer, detoxifier.

Indications: Kidney afflictions (cystitis, nephritis, albuminuria, etc.); water retention; edema; intestinal fermentation.

Verbena (Lemon Verbena, Lippia citriodora, Verbenaceae)

♦ Produced in southern France and North Africa.

♦ Distillation of the branches: The oil is yellowish-green.
♦ Fragrance: Fresh and lemony, similar to lemongrass but more refined.

There is much confusion about verbena oil; many essential oils are improperly called verbena. Indian verbena is a variety of lemongrass, while exotic verbena is *Litsea cubeba*, both plants from the Graminae family (cf. these plants in the Graminae section).

Native to Chile and peru, true lemon verbena is a small bush with an abundant leaf system. The leaves are steam distilled for the production of the oil. The yield is very low, making true lemon verbena oil rather rare and expensive. The world production of the oil is limited and represents only a fraction of the sale of the oil (you can guess where the rest comes from). Lemon verbena is a lovely oil that gives a nice fresh, lemony top note to blends. It is best used in the diffuser.

Medicinal properties: Liver and digestive stimulant; cooling, refreshing, febrifuge; neurovegetative system; calming at low doses.

Indications: Nervousness, insomnia, tachycardia; digestive troubles.

Ylang-Ylang (*Unona odorantissimum*, Anonaceae)

♦ Produced in Reunion, the Comoro Islands, Madagascar, Java, Sumatra, the Philippines.
♦ Fragrance: Sweet, voluptuous, exotic (even sickening for some people).

Ylang-ylang is closely related to cananga (*Canaga odorata*). The two could in fact be the same tree; the slight difference between the essences would then depend on the country of production and the method of distillation.

The distillation of the flowers is a delicate operation, which lasts for days; it yields up to six different qualities, from extra-superior to fifth grade. The "complete" (i.e., the whole oil) should be used for aromatherapy. The oil is yellowish and syrupy and makes a good fragrance fixative.

Ylang-ylang, which means "flower of flowers," is a tree growing up to sixty feet high that produces beautiful yellow flowers. In Indonesia, people spread them on the bed of newly married couples on their wedding night. In the Molucca Islands, People soak ylang-ylang and cucuma flowers in coconut to prepare an ointment called borri-borri that they use for skin care, hair care, and skin disease and to prevent fever. According to R. W. Moncrieff, "ylang-ylang oil soothes and inhibits anger born of frustration."

Supremely exotic, ylang-ylang has the soothing, sedative, slightly euphoric, even lascivious quality of extreme fire and water, the luxurious laziness of tropical islands. It is used especially as a perfume, in baths, for massage, and in cosmetics. It also has a soothing effect on the skin and is recommended for oily skin.

Medicinal properties: Hypotensive; aphrodisiac; antidepressant, sedative, euphoric; antiseptic (for intestinal infections).

Indications: Tachycardia, palpitations; hypertension, hyperpnea; depression, nervous tension, insomnia; impotence, frigidity; skin care.

NINE

The Art of Blending

As I have mentioned before, aromatherapy acts on different levels. On the physical level, essential oils can cure many common diseases. Essential oils also have a profound effect on the energy level, the emotions, and the psyche. More important, aromatherapy has a definitive ludic, Dionysiac dimension to it—it is playful, joyful, lightening, and heartening. Unlike heavy-duty therapy where you have to suffer first to deserve your recovery, enjoyment is part of the aromatic treatment!

Blending is the most creative part of aromatherapy; it is an art. Like any art, it requires a balance of practice and intuition. There are some basic rules, but rules will not create a masterpiece without the proper dose of intuition. Blending is also what makes aromatherapy such a powerful therapeutic tool. You can blend essential oils targeted to treat the specific needs of a specific client, enhancing the effectiveness of your treatments.

To the amateur as well as to the professional, blending is one of the most enjoyable aspects of aromatherapy. It can, in fact, become a very enjoyable hobby. Just as you don't have to be a virtuoso to enjoy violin or piano, you don't have to be a master perfumer to enjoy blending. You might offend the nose of some of your friends once in a while, especially in the beginning, but having fun and learning from your own mistakes is the most important.

Nature has created hundreds of essential oils. In practice, you can readily find on the marketplace fifty to eighty of the most common oils (such as lavender, eucalyptus, lemon, bergamot, cedarwood, or ylang-ylang) and some more exotic and unusual ones (such as cistus, everlasting, lovage, or melissa). While a number of reputable sources offer a wide variety of essential oils, you can use the art of blending to have access to infinite variations.

THE CONCEPT OF SYNERGY

Just like almost anything that deals with life forces, aromatherapy does not abide by the laws of arithmetic. The whole is not the sum of its parts. Two plus two does not necessarily equal four; it might equal three or five, or sometimes even ten! The situation in which the whole is greater than the sum of its parts is called a synergy.

Some essential oils have mutually enhancing powers, while others inhibit each other. A combination of mutually enhancing oils is called a synergy. Synergies help the therapist to be very accurate and precise in the treatment.

Creating synergies is the most important part of blending, requiring a deep understanding of essential oils, a fair amount of experience, and a lot of intuition. Intuition and experience are very important, because synergies are rather context dependent. A given combination of oils might be an excellent synergy for one patient, but totally inappropriate for another.

To create a good synergy, you need to take into account not only the symptoms that you want to treat, but also the underlying causes of the disorder, the biological terrain, and the psychological or emotional factors involved.

All this may sound discouraging to the beginner, but if you follow some basic rules, you will be able to create decent blends.

1. Do not blend more than three or four oils at a time in the beginning; wait until you've gained some experience.

2. Do not blend oils with opposite effects (like a calming and a stimulant). Check thoroughly the properties of the oils that you want to blend and make sure that they complement each other for the particular patient you are treating.

3. A blend has to be pleasant to your patient. This is possibly the most important part of blending. Once you have selected the oils that will be efficient in treating your patient's condition, look at their fragrance compatibility and adjust your blend accordingly.

Below, I have given some basic rules about proportions. I have also provided some basic blends that can be used advantageously for common ailments.

THE PRINCIPLES OF BLENDING

For blending purposes, essential oils are classified into top notes, middle notes, and base notes. A good fragrance composition should harmoniously balance these three categories. When I blend, I use an additional set of classifications: modifiers, enhancers, and equalizers, as well as fixatives.

Fragrance classification is bound to be highly subjective. Different authors might disagree on the classification of certain oils. Although, for most of my presentation, I systematically checked my information against other people's findings, I generally relied upon my own knowledge and experience of the oils to establish the classifications. I encourage you to develop your own categories and classifications as you become more experienced with essential oils and blending. Systems of classification are tools and should be used as such. If you find a system that works better for you, do not hesitate to use it.

Top Notes

Top notes will hit you first in a fragrance. They do not last very long, but they are very important in a blend, because they give the first impression of the blend. Top notes are sharp, penetrating, volatile, extreme, and either cold or hot, but never warm. From a chemical point of view, they are found mostly in the aldehydes and the esters. In the plant, they are found in flowers, leaves, and fruits.

Typical top notes include bergamot, petitgrain, neroli, lemon, lime, orange (all citruses, in fact), lemongrass, peppermint, thyme, cinnamon, and clove (see Table 16). While certain top notes can be used rather liberally (lemon, bergamot, petitgrain), the sharpest ones (cinnamon, cloves, thyme) should be used in very small amounts. Top notes should constitute 20 to 40 percent of your blend. Diffuser blends can use larger amounts of top notes.

Middle Notes

Middle notes give body to your blends; they smooth the sharp edges, round the corners. They are warm, round, soft, and mellow. They are often "blend enhancers" (see below), i.e., oils to add to your blend less for their medicinal properties than for their fragrant qualities. Monoterpene alcohols are typically middle notes. They are mostly found in leaves and herbs.

Typical middle notes are rosewood, geranium, lavender, chamomile, and marjoram (see Table 16). Middle notes usually form the bulk of a blend (40 to 80 percent).

Base Notes

Base notes deepen your blend and increase its lasting effect. Base notes are warm, rich, and mostly pleasant. Most of them have traditional ritual uses. They generally affect the chakras and have deep effects on the mental, emotional, and spiritual planes and on the astral body. When smelled from the bottle, base notes may seem rather faint, but, when applied to the skin, they react strongly and release their power, which lasts for several hours.

Typical base notes are sandalwood, clary sage, frankincense, vanilla, benzoin, cedarwood, and spruce (see Table 16). They are found mostly in woods and gums and are typically sesquiterpenes.

While base notes are not really necessary for a diffuser blend (although they do add depth to it), they are almost mandatory in any preparation to be applied to the skin. They can be used as 10 to 25 percent of a blend.

Fixatives

Even deeper than base notes and often grouped with them, fixatives draw your blend into the skin, giving it roots and permanence. They are necessary for long-lasting effect and are deep, intense, and

Table 16

Top notes	Middle notes	Base notes and fixatives
Bergamot	Rosewood	Cistus (fixative)
Petitgrain	Geranium	Clary sage
Neroli	Lavender and lavandin	Patchouli (fixative)
Lemon	Chamomile	Myrrh (fixative)
Lime	Marjoram	Frankincense
Orange	Champaca leaves	Cedarwood
Other citruses	Palmarosa	Spikenard (fixative)
Lemongrass	Caraway	Sandalwood
Peppermint	Hyssop	Vetiver (fixative)
Thyme	Cardamom	Benzoin
Cinnamon	Coriander	Vanilla
Clove	Elemi	Peru Balsam
	Ginger	Spruce
	Pine	

profound. Some animal fixatives, such as musk or civet, can last for days. Typical fixatives are cistus, myrrh, patchouli, and vetiver (see Table 16).

The first hit of a fixative is not necessarily very pleasant (musk or civet are definitively obnoxious, while patchouli is unpleasant to many people and vetiver or cistus may seem weird), but no decent perfume could be made without them. Fixatives should be used sparingly, to avoid overpowering the blend (they rarely account for more than 5 percent of any blend). They are found in roots and gums and are sesquiterpenes or diterpenes.

Oils with More Than One Note

Essential oils have rather complex chemical compositions, which means that many oils have notes in several categories. Certain oils even cover the whole spectrum from top note to base note. This is the case of ylang-ylang, jasmine, osmanthus, or tuberose (with a predominance in the middle and base notes), champaca flowers, and rose (with a predominance in the top and middle notes). Neroli has most of its notes in the top, but also has a fair amount of middle notes. It is not surprising that such well-balanced oils are the most pleasant that nature has to offer. They can, in fact, be used by themselves as perfumes.

Blend Equalizers

Blend equalizers are the oils that help you get rid of sharp edges. They fill the gaps, help your blend flow harmoniously, and control the intensity of your most active ingredients.

Most of the blend equalizers are context dependent—they perform better with certain types of blends. Rosewood, champaca flowers, and wild Spanish marjoram are universal equalizers, while orange and tangerine are great with other citruses (neroli, petitgrain, bergamot), spices (clove, cinnamon, nutmeg), and floral fragrances (ylang-ylang, jasmine, rose, geranium). Fir and pine greatly improve blends of myrtaceae or coniferae. (See Table 17.)

The main purpose of blend equalizers is to hold your blend together while having little effect on its distinctive personality. They can be used in fairly large amounts (up to 50 percent), especially in those blends where you need to use some of the sharpest oils. Blend equalizers can also be used advantageously with the most precious oils (such as rose, jasmine, neroli, or melissa).

Blend Modifiers (or Personifiers)

Blend modifiers are generally the most intense fragrances. They can greatly affect the overall fragrant quality of your blend, even when used in amounts as small as a fraction of 1 percent. They are found at each end of the spectrum and are responsible for the sharp edges or deep roots of a blend. They also give your blend its very special kick, contributing to its distinctive personality (but an extra drop or two might kill it). If your blend is rather flat and uninteresting, you can, at your own risk, add such an oil—drop by drop, please!

Typical blend modifiers are clove, cinnamon, peppermint, thyme, blue chamomile, cistus, and patchouli (see Table 17). Blend modifiers should be used sparingly (never more than 2 or 3 percent).

Table 17

Blend equalizers	Blend modifiers	Blend enhancers	
Rosewood	Clove	Bergamot	Palmarosa
Marjoram	Cinnamon	Cedarwood	Sandalwood
Orange	Peppermint	Geranium	Spruce
Tangerine	Thyme	Clary sage	Ylang-ylang
Fir	Blue chamomile	Lavender	Jasmine
Pine	Cistus	Lemon	Rose
Champaca leaves	Patchouli	Lime	Neroli
Petitgrain		Champaca flowers	Myrrh
		Litsea cubeba	Osmanthus

Blend Enhancers

Between the modifiers and the equalizers we find the enhancers. Enhancers have a pleasant fragrance by themselves. They have enough personality to modify your blend and give it a personal touch, without overpowering it, as long as they are used in reasonable amounts.

Bergamot, cedarwood, geranium, clary sage, lavender, lemon, lime, litsea cubeba, palmarosa, sandalwood, spruce, ylang-ylang, and, for the precious oils, jasmine, rose, neroli, and myrrh belong to this category (see Table 17). Oils like cajeput, eucalyptus, niaouli, and rosemary could also be considered enhancers, although they are best used in blends for inhalation (diffuser, sauna, steam room, etc.). Enhancers may amount to up to 50 percent of your blend, although each individual oil will rarely account for more than 15 percent of the blend.

Natural Extenders

Some essential oils, such as rose, jasmine, or neroli are very expensive, and whenever you use them in a blend you want to make sure that their fragrance is not wasted. For instance, I do not recommend blending neroli and red thyme. Red thyme would totally overpower and destroy the neroli. Instead, you want to find essential oils that are as compatible as possible with neroli from an olfactory point of view. Natural extenders are the oils used with the most expensive and precious oils to make affordable blends that respect the notes of the precious oils. (See Table 18.)

Further Fragrance Classifications

Many different classifications of fragrances have been created for blending purposes. The most commonly used, in addition to the top, middle, and base notes, is a more descriptive classification into floral, fruity, green, balsamic, woody, etc. The classification can be refined at will. You may add further notes for your own use.

Here again, many oils are a combination of several notes. For example, lime and lemon are fruity and green. Champaca flower oil has a fruity apricot-like note with a dominance of floral, jasmine-like fragrance. Lavender combines floral and herbal. Clary sage is musty and floral.

Table 18

Precious oil	Extender
Neroli	Petitgrain, bergamot, tangerine
Rose	Geranium, palmarosa, rosewood
Jasmine	Champaca flowers, ylang-ylang, petitgrain
Champaca flowers	Ylang-ylang, petitgrain
Vanilla	Benzoin, Peru balsam
Sandalwood	Spruce, cedarwood

Bergamot is fruity with green and floral notes. Cinnamon is sweet and spicy. Rosemary is herbal and balsamic. The classification here is bound to be even more subjective than the two former classifications already described.

Table 19 describes the most frequently used notes and gives some guidelines to blending proportions, as well as to mixing various notes. The oil names in italic are those for which the described note is the dominant note.

Table 19

Note	*Blending guidelines*	*Essential oils*
Floral	Usually expensive—the amount to use will be limited by your budget. Blends well with woody, fruity, sweet, vanilla-y, and musty notes, as well as some green notes and some herbal notes. Wasted in balsamic and anise-y notes.	*Rose, neroli, jasmine, ylang-ylang, tuberose, mimosa, osmanthus, champaca flowers, geranium,* palmarosa, lavender, bergamot, petitgrain
Fruity	Inexpensive and easy to blend—can be used in any proportion. Does not blend very well with woods and very poorly with balsamics and anise.	*Orange, tangerine, lemon,* lime, grapefruit, bergamot, petitgrain, champaca flowers (apricot note), blue chamomile (apple note)
Green	Blends well with any oil. Use in small amounts (1 to 10 percent), especially the mints.	*Peppermint, spearmint, mentha arvensis, lime,* lemon, petitgrain, *citronella, lemongrass, Litsea cubeba, melissa, lemon verbena,* bergamot, ginger
Herbal	Blends well with balsamics and woods. Use with caution with flowers.	*Most labiatae (basil, all sages, hyssop, lavender, marjoram, rosemary, lemon thyme),* angelica, caraway, cardamom, *all chamomiles,* coriander, everlasting, ginger, palmarosa
Balsamic	Gives a very medicinal feel to any blend. Destroys florals. Does not do well with fruits. Best used with woods and herbals.	*Myrtaceae (Eucalyptus, niaouli, cajeput, myrtle, tea tree),* birch, cypress, *pine, fir,* rosemary, *spike,* juniper, *therebentine*
Spicy	Use very small amounts (0.5 to 5 percent). Adds an interesting note to any blend. Can also make or break a blend.	*Clove, bay, cinnamon leaf and bark,* nutmeg, pepper, basil eugenol, *oregano, red thyme, savory*

Table 19 (continued)

Note	Blending guidelines	Essential oils
Woody	Blends well with any oil to make the warm, deep heart of the blend (10 to 20 percent).	*Cedarwood, sandalwood, spruce, frankincense,* cypress, juniper
Musty, earthy	Gives depth and roots to any blend. Use in 3 to 10 percent amount.	*Cistus,* clary sage, elemi, *frankincense, myrrh, mugwort, patchouli, vetiver,* angelica
Exotic, sensual, oriental	Can be overused. Expensive, but worth every penny. Indulge without excess or may be sickening.	*Jasmine, ylang-ylang, champaca flowers, tuberose, osmanthus, sandalwood, patchouli*
Sweet	Blends with any oils, to give warmth and roundness. A fairly large amount of the lighter ones can be used.	*Champaca leaves, marjoram, rosewood,* cardamom, coriander, cinnamon bark, spruce, *tangerine, vanilla, benzoin, Peru balsam*
Anise-y	Difficult to use in blending. Use only in small amounts (10 percent maximum).	*Aniseed, basil, star anise,* caraway, coriander, *fennel, tarragon*
Vanilla-y	Blends with any oil for its characteristic touch but can be overpowering. Use for 2 to 5 percent of blend (maximum 10 percent).	*Vanilla, benzoin, Peru balsam*

Blending guidelines

Fragrance is a great stimulant of the imagination. Therefore, I always encourage people to use images when creating a blend. One of my favorite images for blend creation is that of a human assembly, a social event. Are you coordinating a work group, throwing a lavish party, having a neighborhood barbecue, or preparing for an intimate, romantic evening?

When creating a blend, first look at the purpose of the blend, its use. A blend to fight an infection will be very different from one to soothe emotional wounds or to relieve stress. An infection-fighting blend will be built like a small commando of very efficient no-nonsense soldiers. You want to get the job done, as quickly and cleanly as possible. Your main concern is that the purpose be clear and that all oils used work in a very disciplined way toward the same goal. Fragrance is totally secondary.

For emotional problems on the other hand, fragrance is of the utmost importance, and you will need to carefully and skillfully build your blend to produce a pleasant one.

1) It is important to have a clearly defined purpose when creating a blend. Most beginners try to cure everything with one single blend. Everytime I give a seminar on blending, a few students come up with a blend to cure menopause, arthritis, asthma, cellulitis, spleen problems, and stress, plus balance all the chakras in one single shot. This is the best recipe for failure and represents a misunderstanding of the concept of synergy. Essential oils can be used in many ways and applied to many areas of the body. Do not try to treat the lungs and the kidneys with the same blend. Instead, create a blend for each area that you want to address. Create each blend so that it attacks the problem from different angles, treating when possible the causes as well as the symptoms.

2) Once you determine the purpose of your blend, you have to decide how you are going to use it: through inhalation with a diffuser, applied to the body in massage, bath, compress, or lotion, in skin care preparations, or in special preparations such as personal blends or perfume oils. Lungs are best treated with diffusers or compresses. Emotional issues are best treated with diffusers. Energy issues can be a combination of diffusers and body applications. Physical conditions should be treated through body applications. Be realistic: remember, for example, that inhalation is a useless route for treating cellulite or arthritis.

The more physical the problem, the less important the fragrance of the blend. You should still always try to avoid aromatic disasters. Antiseptic, analgesic, or anti-cellulite blends need to do the job, whatever it takes. Live-on blends (lotions, body oils) should be more sophisticated than the take-off blends (bath products, compresses, masks, cleansers). Skin care blends, especially those that are applied at the end of the skin care session (such as toners, creams, and lotions) should have as nice a fragrance as possible—the nose is right in the middle of the face.

Blends for emotional problems should be as pleasant as possible. For personal blends and perfume oil, sophistication is mandatory. Personal blends are usually created to address deep emotional issues and are used on pressure points and chakras or sniffed directly from the bottle throughout the day. Such blends require a good balance of top, middle, and base notes.

3) The next step will be to define the theme of the blend, the star of the blend. Are you going to invite a royalty, a celebrity, such as rose, neroli, jasmine, tuberose, or mimosa, to your gathering? If so, make sure that you don't spoil the party by inviting some rogue oils such as red thyme, savory, clove, or the balsamics. You may use them in very small amounts, just as body guards watching the doors, but keep them well under 5 percent. Also, do not invite too many celebrities to the same party. Not only do they run up your bill quite fast, they also have strong personalities and bicker, or they pout and disappear for the rest of the party. My advice to the beginner is to use the stars only when you really need them and only one at a time, until you figure out who gets along with whom.

Of course, not every blend needs a celebrity. It does not make sense to bring rose or jasmine to treat digestive or intestinal problems. In general, the precious oils are kept for emotional problems or for leave-on types of preparations, especially those applied to the face.

If you choose a celebrity, a precious oil, make sure it is properly surrounded. The entourage should enhance the fragrance of the precious oil. Use the corresponding extenders. Avoid the clashes such as the balsamics with the florals. Use spices sparingly and cautiously. Finally, find a good balance of top, middle, and base. I have found that a small amount of cistus (2 to 4 percent), brings a deep, rich, musk-like base touch to floral blends, especially when combined with 5 to 10 percent of sandalwood.

Precious oils, if treated properly, will add a nice personality to your blend; conversely, without precious oils a blend may lack personality. Blends that use a lot of equalizers for instance (such as marjoram, rosewood, orange, or tangerine), might end up being rather flat and boring, like a gathering of nice, decent but rather shy people. Such blends can be greatly enhanced by the modifiers, such as spices and vanilla-y notes.

Unscented Bases and Carrier Oils for Preparations

Once you have mixed your blend, you will use it straight only for inhalation (diffuser, sauna, steam room). For most other purposes, you will need to add some of your blend to a carrier oil or an unscented base. Carrier oils and unscented bases are now readily available; refer to the Resource Guide (unscented products can be purchased by those interested in making their own preparations). Tables 20–34, at the end of this chapter, give proper dosages for the most common preparations.

The Carrier Oils

Many vegetable oils can be used as carriers for your aromatherapy preparations. I classify them into bases and active additives, which will be active ingredients in your preparation. They are used in small amounts for their medicinal and skin rejuvenation or skin protection properties.

The Bases

Apricot kernel oil: A fine and nourishing oil, especially recommended for skin care.

Avocado oil: Used mainly in skin care for its nourishing and restorative properties and its high vitamin content.

Canola: Low erucic acid rapeseed oil, expressed from the seeds of *Brassica campestris.* It is very light and odorless and penetrates easily, which makes it a good massage oil base. Its high linoleic acid content prevents rancidity. Low in polyunsaturates, canola oil is good for cooking in that it helps with high cholesterol problems.

Grapeseed oil: The refined oil obtained by pressing numerous varieties of grape seeds. It is a highly polyunsaturated triglyceride oil. A fairly new oil on the American market, it is becoming very popular among beauticians and massage therapists. Very light and odorless, it absorbs easily through the skin. It cleanses, tones, and is widely used in hypoallergenic products as a great emollient film former on skin and hair.

Hazelnut oil: The oil obtained from the nuts of various species of the hazelnut tree, genus *Corylus*. Highly concentrated in Vitamin E, it provides deep skin nourishment and moisturizing action and improves cutaneous circulation. It is noncomedogenic and astringent, tightens the pores, and helps to normalize sebaceous secretions; therefore it is recommended for oily and combination skin.

Jojoba oil: Expressed or extracted from the bean-like seed of the desert shrub *Simmondsia chinensis*. Used by the Native American Indians, jojoba oil is actually a wax; therefore it does not become rancid, which makes it the ideal carrier for perfume oils. Highly emollient, it contains nutrients that feed the skin and regulate its functions. It softens and moisturizes skin, hair, and fingernails. It permeates the stratum corneum, skin, and hair follicles and is very soothing after sun exposure. Some believe that it tends to clog the pores, while others find it very emollient and nourishing for the skin. It is also excellent for hair care (recommended for hair oil base).

Sesame oil: Sun protection. Sesamol and sesamoline are natural antioxidants (found only in the virgin cold-pressed oil).

Sweet almond oil: The triglyceride oil expressed from the ripe seed kernels of the almond tree, *Prunus amygdalus dulcis* or *communis*. It is a light, nondrying oil and a natural emollient oil for skin and hair. Since it does not have a good shelf life, keep it in glass and move to smaller containers as the amount you have decreases.

The Active Additives

Squalane: A saturated branched chain hydrocarbon derived from olives. Occurring naturally in the skin and found in human sebum, it has high affinity with the skin and its natural lipids. It helps the skin act as a barrier and helps avoid transepidermal water loss (TEWL).

Helio-carrot or carrot oil: Obtained from the carrots that are the roots of the *Daucus carota sativa*. Rich in vitamin A, it has cell-regenerating properties. It is recommended before and after sun exposure to help maintain suntan and gives firmness to the skin while helping to prevent wrinkles.

Borage oil: Obtained from the seeds of *Borago officinalis* and very popular in Europe for skin care. It has one of the highest gamma linoleic acid (GLA) contents (19 to 24 percent). GLA, an essential fatty acid, is at the origin of one class of prostaglandin. It increases the protecting function of skin cells, reinforces the skin as a protecting membrane, and is essential for the function and lipid synthesis of the keratinosomes. Research has demonstrated that GLA applied to the skin is incorporated into the phospholipid molecules, which include essential fatty acids known as omega-3 and omega-6 (alpha-linoleic acid). They are essential for health because of their contribution to critical metabolic functions like fingernails, skin, and hair production; visual function; adrenal function (stress); and sperm formation. GLA helps restore the intercellular moisture barrier in the stratum corneum and reduces transepidermal water loss. It moisturizes the skin from within, providing nonocclusive moisturization. Deficiency in GLA increases TEWL, causing severe dryness. Borage oil is recommended in face oils for its rejuvenative power. It should be refrigerated.

Evening primrose: The oil obtained from *Oenothera biennis* or *Oenothera lamarckensi.* It is an expensive oil, rich in gamma-linoleic acid (13 to 15 percent), and therefore excellent for skin care (cf. borage oil). I recommend adding small amounts to a face oil. This oil, being highly unsaturated, easily becomes rancid and should be refrigerated.

Rosa musceta: From the Chilean rosehip seeds. This is another oil with a high gamma-linoleic acid content. It is an emollient, nourishing, tissue regenerator and is recommended for face oils.

Wheatgerm oil: Rich in vitamins E, A, and B. Its antioxidant properties make it useful in oil base preparations to prevent rancidity. It helps regenerate tissues and promotes skin elasticity. Being rather heavy and having a fairly strong odor, it is used in small amounts in the carrier.

Vitamin E (tocopherol): An organic heterocyclic compound derived from soy. It protects the skin from ultraviolet radiation. It is an excellent natural antioxidant and free-radical scavenger. Free radicals are responsible for the aging process and are caused by numerous environmental factors (pollution, gas pipes, air conditioning, smoking).

Other Carriers: Emulsifiers

Essential oils do not mix directly with water. Emulsifiers are necessary to mix oil and water and therefore needed every time we want to incorporate essential oils into water. Emulsifiers are molecules with two radicals, one hydrophile (likes water) and one lipophile (likes oil). Several suppliers, such as Aroma Véra, offer emulsifiers or essential oil solubilizers (see Appendix III).

Suggested base for a face oil in milliliters (thirty-milliliter to one-ounce preparation):

Hazelnut oil: 8
Squalene: 8
Jojoba: 8
Helio-carrot: 3
Evening primrose, borage, or rosa musceta (or a combination of all): 2
Vitamin E: 1

Suggested base for a massage oil in ounces (four-ounce preparation):

Canola oil: 2
Grapeseed oil: 1.5
Wheatgerm oil: 0.5

The Problem of Rancidity

Except for jojoba (which is a wax), any vegetable oil will eventually oxidize and become rancid. Keep your bases in tightly closed dark bottles and store them in a cool place (keep them in your fridge if you use them infrequently). I have noticed that essential oils have antioxidant properties: your aromatherapy preparations will keep longer than the carriers alone. They will have some shelf life, but will still eventually go rancid. If stored properly, any oil base preparation should keep for at least six months.

FORMULAS FOR SOME COMMON AILMENTS

Several manufacturers offer an extensive range of premixed blends for a wide range of indications (refer to Appendix III). I encourage you, however, to prepare your own blends. It adds to the fun and the efficiency of your aromatherapy treatment. Tables 20–34 give you some guidelines. Once you become more acquainted with the power of the oils, you will be able to create your own blends.

Table 20
Formulas for Accumulation and Elimination of Toxins and Related Problems

Accumulation and elimination problems		Cellulitis		Obesity and water retention	
Oil	%	Oil	%	Oil	%
Angelica root	5	Fennel	10	Fennel	10
Caraway seeds	5	Grapefruit	15	Grapefruit	25
Carrot seed	5	Thyme, red	5	Lemon	20
Coriander seeds	5	Cypress	10	Lime	10
Fennel	15	Birch	10	Orange	10
Juniper	15	Geranium	10	Juniper	10
Birch	20	Lemon	20	Thyme, red	5
Grapefruit	30	Rosemary	20	Birch	10

Application methods: Bath, compress, massage, friction/unguent, body wrap.

Complementary treatments
   Drink a lot of liquids (herb teas or water), including one glass, first thing in the morning.
   Cut down on meat, carbohydrates, milk products, salt.
   Eat a lot of raw or steamed vegetables (especially roots).
   Exercise.
   Cellulitis: Massage, frictions, cold showers.
   Obesity: Emotional support or psychotherapy might be necessary.
   Build up self-esteem. Be good to yourself.

Table 21
The Feminine Cycle

Amenorrhoea, dismenorrhoea		Feminine reproductive system (regulation)		Frigidity	
Oil	%	Oil	%	Oil	%
Marjoram	20	Chamomile, Roman	5	Clary sage	5
Chamomile, Roman	10	Chamomile, German	5	Jasmine	10
Chamomile, German	10	Clary sage	5	Rose	10
Mugwort	10	Fennel	5	Ylang-ylang	20
Lavender	25	Rose	5	Sandalwood	10
Clary sage	15	Marjoram	40	Tangerine	45
Fennel	10	Lavender	35		

Menopause		Premenstrual syndrome	
Oil	%	Oil	%
Chamomile, Roman	5	Clary sage	10
Chamomile, German	5	Fennel	10
Mugwort	5	Carrot seed	5
Sage	5	Lavender	20
Geranium	10	Marjoram	30
Bergamot	20	Mugwort	5
Lavender	25	Rosewood	20
Jasmine	5		
Ylang-ylang	20		

Application methods: Bath, compress, massage, friction/unguent, douche.

Table 22
Articular and Muscular Problems

Arthritis		Muscular and articular pain		Rheumatism	
Oil	*%*	*Oil*	*%*	*Oil*	*%*
Birch	30	Birch	40	Birch	20
Ginger root	10	Oregano	5	Cajeput	10
Juniper	10	Bay	5	Ginger root	10
Marjoram	20	Pepper	5	Juniper	10
Rosemary	20	Peppermint	20	Rosemary	10
Thyme, red	5	Clove buds	5	Thyme, red	5
Vetiver	5	Nutmeg	10	Marjoram	20
		Rosemary	10	Nutmeg	10
				Pepper	5

Application methods: Bath, compress, massage, poultice, friction/unguent.
Complementary treatments
　　Drink a lot of liquids (herb tea and water).
　　Cut down on salt.
　　Eat raw and steamed vegetables (celery, cabbage, roots).
　　Massage and baths are particularly indicated.
　　Moderate exercise.

Table 23
Respiratory Related Disorders

Bronchitis		Colds		Respiratory system	
Oil	*%*	*Oil*	*%*	*Oil*	*%*
Eucalyptus	30	Pine	20	Cajeput	20
Fir	20	Spruce	20	Eucalyptus	20
Hyssop	10	Therebentine	20	Fir	20
Lavender	10	Eucalyptus	20	Lavender	20
Myrtle	10	Lavender	20	Niaouli	10
Pine	10			Peppermint	10
Spruce	10				

Respiratory weakness		Sinusitis	
Oil	*%*	*Oil*	*%*
Fir	40	Eucalyptus	40
Pine	40	Lavender	40
Spruce	30	Peppermint	20

Application methods: Diffuser, compress, massage, friction/unguent.
Complementary treatments
　　Breathing exercises, walks in forest or along beaches.
　　Diet: cut down on carbohydrates and dairy products.

Table 24
Blood Circulation

Bruises		Circulation (varicosis, cold feet, tired legs)	
Oil	%	Oil	%
Everlasting	20	Benzoin resinoid	15
Geranium	20	Cinnamon leaf	5
Lavender	50	Cypress	20
Chamomile, blue	10	Lemon	30
		Oregano	10
		Geranium	20

Application methods

Compress	Bath
Lotion	Compress
Friction/unguent	Massage
	Friction/unguent
	Body wrap

Table 25
Digestion

Digestive system		Fatigue, anemia, convalescence	
Oil	%	Oil	%
Bergamot	10	Basil	10
Caraway seeds	5	Cardamom	10
Cardamom	5	Ginger root	10
Coriander seeds	5	Juniper	5
Fennel	5	Nutmeg	10
Ginger root	5	Peppermint	10
Grapefruit	20	Rosemary	30
Lemon	25	Spearmint	15
Orange	20		
Tangerine	20		

Application methods

Bath	Bath
Massage	Diffuser
Friction/unguent	Massage
	Friction/unguent

Table 26
Headaches and Migraines

Headaches		Migraines		Digestive origin of migraines	
Oil	*%*	*Oil*	*%*	*Oil*	*%*
Chamomile, Roman	10	Lavender	30	Basil	10
Peppermint	20	Marjoram	30	Chamomile, Roman	10
Rosewood	40	Melissa	10	Ginger root	10
Spearmint	10	Peppermint	20	Lavender	20
Lavender	20	Spearmint	10	Marjoram	30
				Peppermint	20
				Spearmint	10

Application methods: Compress, diffuser, massage, friction/unguent.
Complementary treatments
    Relaxation, breathing exercises.
    Avoid heavy food (meat, eggs, rich sauces, etc).
    Physical exercise.

Table 27
Impotence

Oriental blend		Spicy blend	
Oil	*%*	*Oil*	*%*
Clary sage	10	Clary sage	10
Jasmine	20	Ginger root	10
Sandalwood mysore	20	Nutmeg	10
Ylang-ylang	20	Pepper	10
Champaca leaves	20	Peppermint	10
Vetiver	5	Sandalwood mysore	20
Cistus	5	Ylang-ylang	20
		Vetiver	10

Application methods: Bath, compress, massage, friction/unguent.
Complementary treatments
    Relaxation, exercise: avoid stress.
    Eat proteins and spicy, earthy food (meat may be recommended).
    Avoid alcohol excess.

Table 28
Infectious Diseases and Epidemics

Oil	%
Eucalyptus	30
Lavender	20
Myrtle	20
Peppermint	10
Tea tree	10
Thyme, red	10

Application methods: Bath, compress, diffuser, massage, friction/unguent.

Table 29
Insect Repellants

Fleas		Mosquitos		Moths	
Oil	%	Oil	%	Oil	%
Lavender	30	Citronella	25	Lavender	50
Lavandin	30	Geranium	25	Lavandin	50
Pennyroyal	20	Lemongrass	25		
Spike	20	Pennyroyal	25		

Application methods

Fleas	Mosquitos	Moths
Diffuser	Diffuser	Diffuser
Friction/unguent	Lotion	Place an aromatic
Sprinkle in infested areas	Friction/unguent	pottery in drawer

Table 30
Insomnia

Oil	%	Oil	%
Chamomile, Roman	10	Marjoram	20
Lavender	20	Neroli	20
Marjoram	20	Orange	15
Orange	15	Tangerine	15
Tangerine	15	Ylang-ylang	20
Ylang-ylang	10	Spikenard	10
Spikenard	10		

Application methods: Baths, diffuser, massage.
Complementary treatments
　　Relaxation, yoga, breathing exercise.
　　Physical exercise (work out).
　　Avoid stress.
　　Balance your diet: Vitamins and minerals are advised.

Table 31
Emotional Problems, Stress, and Brain Stimulation
(for Use in Diffuser, Massage, and Bath)

Anxiety		Depression			
		Indulging formula		*Uplifting formula*	
Oil	%	Oil	%	Oil	%
Benzoin resinoid	10	Bergamot	10	Lemon	10
Bergamot	10	Geranium	15	Lime	20
Clary sage	10	Jasmine	10	Melissa	10
Jasmine	10	Petitgrain	10	Peppermint	10
Lemon	10	Rose	5	Petitgrain	20
Patchouli	10	Sandalwood mysore	10	Rosemary	20
Petitgrain	20	Ylang-ylang	20	Thyme, lemon	10
Rosewood	20	Rosewood	20		

Complementary treatments
　　Relax, be good to yourself, treat yourself.
　　Start a new project: Physical exercise is strongly recommended.
　　Balance your diet: Vitamins and minerals are suggested.

Table 31 (continued)

Emotional shock, grief		*Neurasthenia*		*Sadness*	
Oil	*%*	*Oil*	*%*	*Oil*	*%*
Melissa	10	Lavender	20	Benzoin resinoid	20
Neroli	10	Melissa	10	Rosewood	40
Rose	10	Patchouli	10	Jasmine	10
Tangerine	60	Rosemary	40	Rose	10
Sandalwood	10	Thyme, lemon	20	Ylang-ylang	20

Complementary treatments
Yoga, meditation.
Psychotherapy and emotional support are strongly advised.

Energy		*Memory (poor)*		*Mental fatigue*	
Oil	*%*	*Oil*	*%*	*Oil*	*%*
Benzoin resinoid	10	Basil	10	Basil	20
Cedarwood	20	Clove buds	10	Cardamom	20
Clary sage	10	Ginger root	10	Ginger root	20
Fir	30	Juniper	10	Peppermint	20
Spruce	30	Petitgrain	30	Rosemary	20
		Rosemary	30		

Complementary treatments
Vitamins and minerals.
Reduce stress.
Balance diet (eat enough protein).

Nervous tension, nervousness		*Stress*		*Tension*	
Oil	*%*	*Oil*	*%*	*Oil*	*%*
Geranium	10	Cedarwood	20	Clary sage	20
Lavender	10	Clary sage	20	Marjoram	20
Marjoram	20	Fir	20	Lavender	20
Melissa	10	Pine	20	Ylang-ylang	20
Neroli	10	Spruce	20	Petitgrain	20
Tangerine	40	Ylang-ylang	20		
Ylang-ylang	10				

Complementary treatments
Relaxation (yoga or meditation).
Massage and baths are strongly recommended.

Table 32
Skin Care Formulas Used in Facials, Masks, Compresses, Lotions, Facial and Body Oils, and Body Wraps

Acne		*Dermatitis*		*Wrinkles*	
Oil	*%*	*Oil*	*%*	*Oil*	*%*
Bergamot	10	Cedarwood	10	Clary sage	5
Juniper	5	Juniper	5	Frankincense	5
Lavender	10	Lavender	10	Myrrh	5
Palmarosa	20	*Litsea cubeba*	10	Patchouli	5
Peppermint	5	Palmarosa	20	Rose	10
Rosemary	10	Peppermint	10	Rosemary	20
Sandalwood mysore	10	Rosewood	20	Rosewood	30
Thyme, lemon	30	Thyme, lemon	15	Geranium	20

Dry skin		*Oily skin*		*Sensitive skin*	
Oil	*%*	*Oil*	*%*	*Oil*	*%*
Clary sage	10	Clary sage	10	Chamomile, Roman	5
Jasmine	10	Ylang-ylang	20	Everlasting	5
Palmarosa	30	Lavender	10	Jasmine	10
Rosemary	20	Lemon	30	Neroli	10
Rose	10	Geranium	20	Rose	10
Sandalwood	20	Frankincense	10	Rosewood	60

Table 33
Hair Care Formulas Used in Shampoos, Rinses, Lotions, and Hair Oils

Oily hair		*Hair loss (growth)*		*Dandruff*	
Oil	*%*	*Oil*	*%*	*Oil*	*%*
Cedarwood	25	Bay	20	Cedarwood	20
Sage	25	Clary sage	10	Patchouli	20
Lemongrass	25	Ylang-ylang	20	Rosemary	20
Rosemary	25	Cedarwood	20	Sage	20
		Rosemary	20	Tea tree	20
		Sage	10		

Table 34
Chakra and Energy Formulas Used in Unguent, Diffuser, and Massage

Crown chakra		Third eye		Heat chakra	
Oil	%	Oil	%	Oil	%
Benzoin resinoid	10	Cistus	5	Benzoin resinoid	40
Cistus	5	Frankincense	5	Melissa	10
Frankincense	5	Myrrh	10	Neroli	30
Myrrh	10	Sandalwood mysore	20	Rose	20
Sandalwood mysore	20	Spruce	50		
Spruce	40	Mugwort	10		
Rose	10				

Solar plexus		Sexual chakra		Root chakra	
Oil	%	Oil	%	Oil	%
Rosemary	30	Jasmine	20	Pepper	40
Sage	20	Ylang-ylang	30	Vetiver	30
Lemon	30	Sandalwood	20	Frankincense	30
Clove	10	Tangerine	30		
Juniper	10				

Yoga, meditation, rituals		Astral bodies		Psychic centers	
Oil	%	Oil	%	Oil	%
Cedarwood	20	Lavender	20	Cistus	5
Cistus	5	Marjoram	30	Elemi	10
Fir	30	Melissa	10	Frankincense	10
Myrrh	5	Patchouli	10	Myrrh	10
Sandalwood mysore	15	Rosemary	20	Cedarwood	25
Spruce	25	Thyme, lemon	10	Spruce	40

APPENDIX I

Essential Oils
Reference Table

This table has been created to help you find rapidly the information that you may need in your daily practice. It might seem overwhelming at first glance, but I hope you find it comprehensive and practical. Many oils listed here cannot easily be found in any other book. I also differentiate between the varieties of the same species (such as chamomiles or the chemotypes of thyme). Since there are a few hundred essential oils, some have been left out. Still, I cover all the common oils plus all those that present some therapeutic interest and can be found on the market.

The following codes represent suggested uses of oils for specific conditions:

D	Diffuser
M	Massage
B	Bath
F	Facial masks
C	Compresses
L	Lotions
O	Oil for face or body
U	Unguents.

The power of the oil is indicated with regard to the specific condition on a scale from 1 to 5.

Essential Oils Reference Table

Plant name (*Genus species/ family*)	Property	Indication	Use	Power
Angelica root (*Angelica archangelica/* Umbelliferae)	Medicinal			
	Cleanser, depurative, drainer	Accumulation (toxins, fluids)	MBFCLO	4
	Stimulant digestive	Digestive problems, migraine	DCU	3
	Revitalizing, stimulant	Anemia, asthenia, anorexia convalescence, rachitism	DMB	4
	Carminative	Aerophagia	MBC	3
	Cleanser, depurative, drainer	Gout	MCU	3
	Antispasmodic	Digestive spasms	MBCU	3
Aniseed (*Pimpinella anisum/* Umbelliferae)	Medicinal			
	Carminative	Aerophagia	MBC	4
	Digestive stimulant	Digestive problems, migraine	DCU	4
	Antispasmodic	Digestive spasms	MBCU	3
	Galactagogue	Insufficient milk	MBCU	3
	Aphrodisiac	Frigidity, impotence	MBCU	2
Basil (*Ocymum basilicum/* Labiatae)	Medicinal			
	Antiseptic (intestinal)	Intestinal infections	MCU	3
	Stimulant	Vital centers	DMBU	4
	Cephalic	Migraine	DCU	4
	Antispasmodic, stomachic	Dyspepsia, gastric spasms	MCU	3
	Facilitates birth and nursing	Nursing, pregnancy	DMBU	2
	Mind, emotion, psyche			
	Stimulant	Memory (poor), neurovegetative system	DMBU	4
	Tonic (nervous)	Nervous fatigue, intellectual, mental fatigue, mental strain	DMBU	4
	Contraindications			
	Stupefying	High doses		2
Bay (*Pimenta racemosa/* Myrtaceae)	Body and skin care			
	Scalp stimulant	Hair growth	LO	4
	Medicinal			
	Antiseptic, stimulant	Respiratory system	DMBCU	3
	Antiseptic	Infectious diseases	DMBCU	3
	Analgesic, antineuralgic	Pain (muscular and articular), neuralgia	MBCU	3
Benzoin resinoid (*Styrax benzoin/* Styraceae)	Body and skin care			
	Rejuvenating, stimulant	Skin elasticity	FCLOU	2
	Medicinal			
	Appeasing, balancing	Energy inbalance	DMB	4

Essential Oils Reference Table (continued)

Plant name (*Genus species/* family)	Property	Indication	Use	Power
	Regulator	Secretions	MBCU	3
	Expectorant	Bronchitis	DMBC	3
	Soothing	Cough, laryngitis	D	3
	Stimulant	Circulation	MBCU	2
	Antiseptic, diuretic	Genitourinary infections, urinary infections	MBC	2
	Healing	Cracked and chapped skin, dermatitis, skin irritation, skin rashes, wounds	CLU	4
	Mind, emotion, psyche			
	Purifier	Drive out evil spirits	DU	3
	Stimulant	Crown chakra, heart chakra	DU	3
	Comforting, euphoric	Anxiety, loneliness, sadness	DMBU	3
	Comforting, uplifting	Exhaustion (psychic and emotional)	DMBU	3
Bergamot (*Citrus bergamia/* Rutaceae)	Body and skin care			
	Antiseptic, vulnerary	Acne, eczema, seborrhea	FCLO	3
	Medicinal			
	Refreshing	Hot climates	DMBLU	3
	Stimulant	Digestive problems	MBC	3
	Balancing	Nervous system	DMBU	4
	Antispasmodic, digestive	Colics, intestinal infections	MCU	3
	Antiseptic, vulnerary	Leukorrhea, vaginal pruritus	MU	3
	Mind, emotion, psyche			
	Antidepressant, uplifting	Anxiety, depression	DMB	4
	Contraindications			
	Increases photosensitivity	Do not apply neat before sun	MFCLOU	3
Birch (*Betula lenta* and *betula nigra/* Betulaceae)	Medicinal			
	Analgesic	Arthritis, pain (muscular and articular), rheumatism	MBCU	4
	Cleanser, depurative, drainer	Accumulation (toxins, fluids), cellulitis, obesity, water retention	MBCU	3
	Diuretic	Cystitis, kidneys	MBCU	4
Cajeput (*Melaleuca leucadendron/* Myrtaceae)	Medicinal			
	Balancing, reequilibrating	Energy inbalance	DMB	3
	Antiseptic, antispasmodic	Respiratory system	DMBCU	5
	Antiseptic	Infectious diseases	DMBCU	4

Essential Oils Reference Table (continued)

Plant name (*Genus species/* family)	Property	Indication	Use	Power
	Antiseptic (urinary)	Cystitis, urethritis, urinary infections	MBC	4
	Balsamic, expectorant	Asthma, bronchitis, tuberculosis	DMBCU	5
	Antineuralgic	Rheumatism	MBCU	3
	Antiseptic (intestinal)	Amebas, diarrhea, dysentery	MB	3
	Analgesic, antiseptic	Earache	U	4
	Antiseptic, expectorant	Sinusitis	DU	5
Caraway seeds (*Carum carvi/* Umbelliferae)	Medicinal			
	Cleanser, depurative, drainer	Accumulation (toxins, fluids)	MBFCLO	3
	Stimulant, digestive stimulant	Digestive problems	MBC	4
	Stimulant general	Energy deficiency	DMB	3
	Carminative	Aerophagia, fermentation	MBC	4
	Antispasmodic	Dyspepsia, migraine, digestive spasms	MBCU	3
	Parasiticide	Scabies	CLU	2
	Diuretic	Kidneys	MBCU	2
	Tissue regenerator	Infected wounds	FCLOU	3
	Stimulant	Glandular system	MBU	2
	Mind, emotion, psyche			
	Tonic (nervous)	Mental fatigue, mental strain	DMBU	3
Cardamom (*Eletteria cardamomum/* Zingiberaceae)	Medicinal			
	Stimulant	Digestive problems	MBC	4
	Aphrodisiac	Impotence	MBCU	3
		Diarrhea	MBCU	3
Carrot seed (*Dauca carota/* Umbelliferae)	Body and skin care			
	Cleanser, depurative, drainer	Dermatitis	MFCLOU	3
	Stimulate elasticity, tonic	Aged skin, skin irritation, skin rashes, wrinkles	FCLO	3
	Medicinal			
	Cleanser, depurative, drainer	Accumulation (toxins, fluids)	MBFCLO	4
	Stimulant general	Energy deficiency	DMB	2
	Revitalizing, stimulant	Anemia, asthenia, anorexia, convalescence, rachitism	DMB	3
	Cleanser, depurative, hepatic	Hepatobiliary disorders	MBCU	4
	Emmenagogue	Amenorrhea, dysmenorrhea, premenstrual syndrome	MBCU	3
	Stimulant	Glandular system	MBU	3

Essential Oils Reference Table (continued)

Plant name (*Genus species/family*)	Property	Indication	Use	Power
Chamomile, blue (*Ormensis multicolis/* Compositae)	Body and skin care			
	Anti-inflammatory, soothing	Acne, dermatitis, eczema, skin care	FCLO	5
	Anti-inflammatory, soothing	Inflamed skin, sensitive skin	FCLO	4
	Medicinal			
	Analgesic, anti-inflammatory	Arthritis, inflamed joints	BCU	4
	Anti-inflammatory, healing, soothing	Abscess, boils, bruises	CLU	4
	Antispasmodic, sedative	Colics, colitis	MCU	3
	Cholagogue, hepatic	Liver and spleen congestion	MCU	3
	Analgesic, anti-inflammatory	Teething pain, toothache	U	3
Chamomile, German (*Chamomilla matricaria/* Compositae)	Body and skin care			
	Anti-inflammatory, soothing	Acne, dermatitis, eczema, skin care	FCLO	3
	Anti-inflammatory, soothing	Inflamed skin, sensitive skin	FCLO	4
	Medicinal			
	Immunostimulant	Leukocyte formation stimulant	DMU	4
	Analgesic, anti-inflammatory	Arthritis, inflamed joints	BCU	4
	Anti-inflammatory, healing, soothing	Abscess, boils	FCLO	4
	Antispasmodic, sedative	Colics, colitis	MCU	4
	Calming, sedative	Headache, insomnia, irritability, migraine	DCU	4
	Emmenagogue	Amenorrhea, dysmenorrhea, menopause	DMBCU	4
	Analgesic	Teething pain, toothache	U	4
	Antianemic	Anemia, asthenia	DMB	4
	Digestive, stomachic	Digestive problems	MBC	4
	Cholagogue, hepatic	Liver, liver and spleen congestion	MCU	4
	Balancing	Feminine reproductive system	DMBCU	4
	Mind, emotion, psyche			
	Appeasing	Anger, tantrum	DMBU	4
Chamomile, mixta (*Anthemis mixta/* Compositae)	Body and skin care			
	Calming, soothing	Sensitive skin	FCLO	4
	Medicinal			
	Antispasmodic, sedative	Colic, colitis	MCU	3
	Calming, sedative	Headache, insomnia, irritability, migraine	DCU	3
	Emmenagogue	Amenorrhea, dysmenorrhea, menopause	DMBCU	3
	Cholagogue, hepatic	Liver and spleen congestion	MCU	3

Essential Oils Reference Table (continued)

Plant name (*Genus species/ family*)	Property	Indication	Use	Power
Chamomile, Roman (*Anthemis nobilis/* Compositae)	Body and skin care			
	Healing, soothing	Abscess, boils, sensitive skin	FCLO	5
	Medicinal			
	Analgesic	Arthritis, inflamed joints	BCU	3
	Antispasmodic, sedative	Colic, colitis	MCU	4
	Calming, sedative	Headache, insomnia, irritability, migraine	DCU	4
	Emmenagogue	Amenorrhea, dysmenorrhea, menopause	DMBCU	4
	Analgesic	Teething pain, toothache	U	4
	Antianemic	Anemia, asthenia	DMB	4
	Digestive, stomachic	Digestive problems	MBC	4
	Immunostimulant	Leukocyte formation stimulant	DMU	4
	Cholagogue, hepatic	Liver, liver and spleen congestion	MCU	4
	Balancing	Feminine reproductive system	DMBCU	4
	Mind, emotion, psyche			
	Realization	Personal growth	DMBU	4
	Appeasing	Anger, oversensitivity, tantrum	DMBU	4
Cedarwood (*Cedrus atlantica/* Confirae)	Body and skin care			
	Antiseptic, fungicidal	Dandruff, hair loss	LO	4
	Antiseborrheic	Oily hair	LO	3
	Medicinal			
	Tonic	Glandular system, nervous system, respiratory system	DMBCU	4
	Antiseptic (urinary)	Cystitis, urinary infections	MBC	3
	Antiseptic, fungicidal	Dermatitis, eczema, fungal infections, ulcers	FCLO	4
	Mind, emotion, psyche			
	Appeasing	Deep relaxation	DMBU	4
	Appeasing, sedative	Anxiety, stress	DMB	3
	Elevating, grounding, opening	Psychic work, yoga meditation, rituals	DU	3
Cinnamon bark (*Cinnamomum zeylanicum/* Lauraceae)	Medicinal			
	Stimulant	Circulation, heart, nervous system	DMBU	4
	Antiseptic	Flu, infectious diseases	DMBCU	5
	Antispasmodic	Spasms	DMBC	2
	Stimulant	Anemia, asthenia, digestive problems	MBC	3

Essential Oils Reference Table (continued)

Plant name (*Genus species/family*)	Property	Indication	Use	Power
	Parasiticide	Lice, scabies	CLU	3
	Aphrodisiac	Impotence	MBCU	2
	Antiseptic	Intestinal infections	MCU	3
	Contractions stimulant	Childbirth	MCU	3
	Contraindications			
	Irritant (skin)	High doses, neat or in high concentration	BFC	3
	Convulsive	High doses		3
Cinnamon leaf (*Cinnamomum zeylanicum/*Lauraceae)	Medicinal			
	Stimulant	Circulation	MBCU	4
	Antiseptic	Infectious diseases	DMBCU	5
	Parasiticide	Lice, scabies	CLU	3
	Antiseptic	Intestinal infections	MCU	3
	Contraindications			
	Irritant (skin)	High doses, neat or in high concentration	BFC	4
	Convulsive	High doses		4
Cistus (*Cistus ladaniferus/*Cistaceae)	Medicinal			
	Diuretic	Urinary infections	MBC	3
	Drying, vulnerary	Ulcers, wounds	CLU	2
	Mind, emotion, psyche			
	Stimulant	Third eye, crown chakra	DU	5
	Stimulant	Psychic centers	DU	5
	Sedative (nervous)	Insomnia, nervousness	DMBU	3
	Elevating, grounding, opening	Psychic work, yoga, meditation, rituals	DU	5
Citronella (*Cymbopogon nardus/*Graminae)	Medicinal			
	Deodorant, deodorizer, purifier	Sanitation, epidemics	D	4
	Insect repellent	Mosquitos	DLU	5
	Deodorant, deodorizer	Bathroom, garbage	D	4
	Stimulant	Digestive problems	MBC	2
	Antiseptic	Infectious diseases	DMBCU	3
Clary sage (*Salvia sclarea/*Labiatae)	Body and skin care			
	Cell regenerator	Aged skin, wrinkles	FCLO	3
	Soothing	Inflamed skin	FCLO	3
	Regulator of seborrhea	Dry skin, oily skin	FCLO	3
	Regulator of seborrhea	Oily skin	LO	3
	Scalp stimulant, stimulant	Hair growth	LO	3

Essential Oils Reference Table (continued)

Plant name (*Genus species/ family*)	Property	Indication	Use	Power
	Medicinal			
	Antispasmodic, emmenagogue	Menstrual cramps, premenstrual syndrome	MBCU	4
	Emmenagogue	Amenorrhea, dysmenorrhea	MBCU	4
	Balancing, tonic	Feminine reproductive system, feminine energy	DMBU	5
	Mind, emotion, psyche			
	Antidepressant, calming	Anxiety, emotional tension, stress, tension	DMBU	2
	Antidepressant, euphoric	Depression, postnatal depression	DMB	4
Clove buds (*Eugenia caryophyllata/* Myrtaceae)	Medicinal			
	Antiseptic, stimulant	Respiratory system	DMBCU	5
	Antiseptic	Infectious diseases	DMBCU	4
	Antiseptic (urinary)	Urinary infections	MBC	4
	Analgesic, antineuralgic	Pain (muscular and articular), neuralgia, toothache	U	5
	Carminative, stomachic	Dyspepsia, fermentations anemia, asthenia, energy deficiency	MBC	4
			DMB	4
	Aphrodisiac	Impotence	MBCU	3
	Antiseptic, cicatrizant	Infected wounds, ulcers	FCLO	3
	Parasiticide	Scabies	CLU	3
	Mind, emotion, psyche			
	Stimulant (intellectual)	Nervous fatigue, intellectual, memory (poor)	DMBU	4
Coriander seeds (*Coriandrum sativum/* Umbelliferae)	Medicinal			
	Cleanser, depurative, drainer	Accumulation (toxins, fluids)	MBFCLO	3
	Stimulant, digestive	Digestive problems	MBC	4
	Revitalizing, stimulant	Anemia, asthenia, convalescence	DMB	4
	Carminative	Aerophagia, flatulence	MBCU	4
	Analgesic, warming	Gout, rheumatism	MBCU	3
	Aperitive, revitalizing	Anorexia	DMB	3
	Antispasmodic	Migraine, digestive spasms	MBCU	3
	Stimulant	Glandular system	MBU	3
Cumin seeds (*Cuminum cymimum* Umbelliferae)	Medicinal			
	Cleanser, depurative, drainer	Accumulation (toxins, fluids)	MBFCLO	3
	Revitalizing, stimulant	Anemia, asthenia, convalescence	DMB	3

Essential Oils Reference Table (continued)

Plant name (*Genus species/ family*)	Property	Indication	Use	Power
	Carminative	Aerophagia, flatulence	MBCU	4
	Antispasmodic	Digestive spasms	MBCU	3
	Digestive	Digestive problems, migraine	DCU	3
	Stimulant	Heart, nervous system	DMBU	3
Cypress, (*Cupressus sempervirens/* Coniferae)	Medicinal			
	Warming	Energy deficiency	DMB	4
	Tonic	Respiratory system	DMBCU	3
	Tonic (circulation)	Cellulitis, circulation	MBCU	5
	Astringent	Edema, water retention	MBCU	5
	Antispasmodic	Asthma, cough, whooping cough	DMC	4
	Antisudorific, deodorant, deodorizer	Perspiration (especially of feet)	MBCLU	4
Elemi (*Canarium luzonicum/* Burseraceae)	Medicinal			
	Cooling, drying, vulnerary	Infected wounds	FCLOU	3
	Regulator	Secretions	MBCU	4
	Balsamic, expectorant	Catarrhal condition	D	2
	Balsamic	Respiratory system	DMBCU	2
	Mind, emotion, psyche			
	Fortifying	Psychic centers	DU	3
Eucalyptus Australiana (*Eucalyptus polybractea/* (Myrtaceae)	Medicinal			
	Balancing, reequilibrating	Energy inbalance	DMB	4
	Antiseptic, stimulant	Respiratory system	DMBCU	5
	Antiseptic	Infectious diseases	DMBCU	4
	Antiseptic (urinary)	Urinary infections	MBC	4
	Balsamic, expectorant	Asthma, bronchitis tuberculosis	DMBCU	5
	Antidiabetic	Diabetes	MB	3
	Antiseptic, expectorant	Sinusitis	DU	5
Eucalyptus citriodora (Myrtaceae)	Medicinal			
	Antiseptic, bactericide	Infectious diseases	DMBCU	3
	Deodorant, deodorizer, disinfectant	Sanitation	D	3
Eucalyptus globulus (Myrtaceae)	Medicinal			
	Balancing, reequilibrating	Energy inbalance	DMB	4
	Antiseptic, stimulant	Respiratory system	DMBCU	5
	Antiseptic	Infectious diseases	DMBCU	4

Essential Oils Reference Table (continued)

Plant name (*Genus species/ family*)	Property	Indication	Use	Power
	Antiseptic (urinary)	Urinary infections	MBC	4
	Balsamic, expectorant	Asthma, bronchitis, tuberculosis	DMBCU	5
	Vermifuge	Ascarides, oxyurids	MBCU	3
	Antidiabetic	Diabetes	MB	3
Everlasting (*Helicrysum italicum/* Compositae)	Body and skin care			
	Anti-inflammatory, soothing	Acne, dermatitis, skin care	FCLO	3
	Anti-inflammatory, soothing	Inflamed skin, sensitive skin	FCLO	4
	Anti-inflammatory, astringent, healing	Hemorrhage, skin irritation	FCLOU	5
	Medicinal			
	Anti-inflammatory, healing, soothing	Abscess, boils	FCLO	4
	Tissue stimulant	Wounds, cuts	CLU	5
	Cholagogue, hepatic	Liver, liver and spleen congestion	MCU	4
Fennel (*Foeniculum vulgare/* Umbelliferae)	Body and skin care			
	Cleanser, detoxifier	Orange-peel skin	MBCU	5
	Medicinal			
	Cleanser, depurative, drainer	Accumulation (toxins, fluids)	MBFCLO	5
	Stimulant, stimulant digestive	Digestive problems	MBC	4
	Revitalizing, stimulant	Anemia, asthenia, rachitism	DMB	4
	Carminative	Aerophagia, flatulence	MBCU	3
	Antispasmodic	Digestive spasms	MBCU	3
	Cleanser, detoxifier	Cellulitis, obesity, orange-peel skin, water retention	MBCU	5
	Regulator	Amenorrhea, dysmenorrhea, feminine reproductive system, premenstrual syndrome	MBCU	4
	Galactagogue	Insufficient milk (nursing), nursing	DMBU	4
	Stimulant	Glandular system, glandular system (estrogen)	MBU	4
	Contraindications			
	Toxic	Young children (under 6)	MBU	2
Fir (*Abies balsamea/* Coniferae)	Medicinal			
	Warming	Respiratory weakness	DMBU	4
	Tonic	Glandular system, nervous system, respiratory system	DMBCU	4

Essential Oils Reference Table (continued)

Plant name (*Genus species/family*)	Property	Indication	Use	Power
	Antiseptic (urinary)	Genitourinary infections, urinary infections	MBC	3
	Antiseptic, expectorant	Asthma, bronchitis	DMBC	4
	Mind, emotion, psyche			
	Elevating, grounding, opening	Psychic work	DU	5
	Elevating, grounding, opening	Third eye, crown chakra	DU	5
	Appeasing, sedative	Anxiety stress	DMB	5
	Elevating, grounding, opening	Yoga, meditation, rituals	DU	5
Frankincense (*Boswellia carteri/* Burseraceae)	Body and skin care			
	Revitalizing, tonic	Aged skin, wrinkles	FCLO	4
	Medicinal			
	Cooling, drying, vulnerary	Infected wounds, inflammations	FCLU	4
	Regulator	Secretions	MBCU	4
	Balsamic, expectorant	Asthma, catarrhal condition, cough	D	3
	Antiseptic (pulmonary)	Lungs	DCU	3
	Mind, emotion, psyche			
	Fortifying	Mind, psychic centers	DU	5
	Stimulant	Third eye, crown chakra	DU	4
Geranium (*Pelargonium graveolens* and *roseum/* Geraniaceae)	Body and skin care			
	Antiseptic, astringent, cell regenerator	Acne, aged skin, dermatitis, oily skin, skin care	FCLO	3
	Medicinal			
	Astringent, hemostatic	Bruises, hemorrhage	CLU	4
	Antiseptic	Infectious diseases	DMBCU	3
	Antidiabetic	Diabetes	MB	3
	Diuretic	Kidney stones, kidneys	MBCU	3
	Adrenal cortex stimulant	Cellulitis, adrenocortical glands, menopause	DMBCU	3
	Insect repellent	Mosquitos	DLU	3
	Astringent	Sore throat, tonsillitis	U	3
	Antiseptic, cytophilactic	Burns, wounds	CLU	3
	Mind, emotion, psyche			
	Stimulant, uplifting	Depression, nervous tension	DMBU	3

Essential Oils Reference Table (continued)

Plant name (*Genus species/family*)	Property	Indication	Use	Power
Ginger root (*Zingiber officinale/* Zingiberaceae)	Medicinal			
	Stimulant	Digestive problems, memory (poor), neurovegetative system, vital centers	DMBU	4
	Stimulant	Digestive problems	MBC	3
	Cephalic	Migraine	DCU	3
	Antispasmodic, stomachic	Dyspepsia, gastric spasms	MCU	3
	Analgesic	Arthritis, rheumatism,	MBCU	3
	Febrifuge	Fever	MBCU	3
	Carminative	Aerophagia, flatulence	MBCU	3
	Aphrodisiac	Impotence	MBCU	3
		Diarrhea	MBCU	3
	Antiseptic, astringent	Sore throat, tonsillitis	U	3
	Mind, emotion, psyche			
	Stimulant	Memory (poor)	DMBU	4
Grapefruit (*Citrus paradisi/* Rutaceae)	Medicinal			
	Stimulant	Digestive problems	MBC	3
	Control of liquid processes	Lymphatic system and secretions, secretions	MBCU	5
	Drainer, lymphatic stimulant	Cellulitis, obesity, water retention	MBCU	5
Hyssop (*Hysopus officinalis/* Labiatae)	Medicinal			
	Stimulant	Respiratory system, vital centers	DMBU	4
	Antispasmodic, balsamic, expectorant	Asthma, bronchitis, catarrhal condition, whooping cough	DMC	5
	Antispasmodic, expectorant	Whooping cough	DMC	5
	Hypertensor	Hypotension	DMCU	4
	Digestive, stomachic	Digestive problems, dyspepsia	MCU	3
	Cicatrizant, vulnerary	Dermatitis, eczema, wounds	CLU	2
Jasmine (*Jasminum officinalis/* Oleaceae)	Body and skin care			
	Moisturizer, soothing	Dry skin, sensitive skin	FCLO	3
	Healing, soothing	Dermatitis	MFCLOU	3
	Medicinal			
	Aphrodisiac	Frigidity, impotence	MBCU	5
	Mind, emotion, psyche			
	Stimulant	Sexual chakra	DMBU	5
	Antidepressant, euphoric	Anxiety, lethargy, menopause, sadness	DMBU	5

Essential Oils Reference Table (continued)

Plant name (*Genus species/ family*)	Property	Indication	Use	Power
	Uplifting	Lack of confidence	DMBU	4
	Antidepressant, euphoric	Depression, postnatal depression	DMB	5
Juniper (*Juniperus communis/* Coniferae)	Body and skin care Cleanser, detoxifier, drainer Medicinal	Acne, dermatitis, eczema	FCLO	4
	Tonic	Glandular system	MBU	4
	Antiseptic (urinary)	Genitourinary infections, urinary infections	MBC	5
	Diuretic, urinary antiseptic	Cystitis, diabetes, oliguria	MBCU	4
	Cleanser, detoxifier, drainer	Accumulation (toxins, fluids), arthritis, rheumatism, uric acid	MBCU	5
	Mind, emotion, psyche Tonic (nervous)	Nervous and intellectual fatigue, memory (poor)	DMBU	4
Lavender (*Lavandula officinalis/* Labiatae)	Body and skin care Antiseptic, cytophilactic	Acne, dermatitis, eczema, oily skin	FCLO	4
	Healing Medicinal	Psoriasis	CLU	3
	Stimulant	Metabolism, respiratory system, vital centers	DMBU	4
	Antiseptic	Blennorrhea, cystitis, infectious diseases	DMBCU	5
	Antiseptic, cytophylactic	Abscess, bruises, burns, wounds	CLU	5
	Antiseptic, antispasmodic	Asthma, bronchitis, catarrhal condition, colds	DMCU	4
	Decongestant	Sinusitis	DU	5
	Calming, cephalic	Headache, migraine	DCU	4
	Calming	Insomnia, nervous tension, palpitations	DMBC	3
	Insect repellent	Fleas, moths	DU	3
	Antispasmodic, emmenagogue	Amenorrhea, dismenorrhea, menopause, premenstrual syndrome	MBCU	3
	Mind, emotion, psyche Appeasing	Astral body	DMBU	4
	Antidepressant, calming	Depression, neaurasthenia	DMB	4
	Anticonvulsive	Convulsions	DMBC	4

Essential Oils Reference Table (continued)

Plant name (*Genus species/* family)	Property	Indication	Use	Power
Lavandin (*Lavandula fragrans delphinensis/* Labiatae)	Medicinal			
	Stimulant	Respiratory system	DMBCU	3
	Antiseptic	Infectious diseases	DMBCU	4
	Antiseptic, cytophilactic	Burns, wounds	CLU	3
	Deodorant, deodorizer, disinfectant	Sanitation, epidemics	D	3
	Insect repellent	Fleas, mosquitos	DLU	3
	Mind, emotion, psyche			
	Appeasing	Astral body	DMBU	3
Lemon (*Citrus limonum/* Rutaceae)	Body and skin care			
	Antiseptic, depurative, lymphatic stimulant	Oily skin, skin care	FCLO	4
	Medicinal			
	Digestive, stimulant	Digestive problems	MBC	4
	Control of liquid processes	Lymphatic system and secretions, secretions	MBCU	4
	Hepatobiliary stimulant	Gall bladder congestion, liver	MCU	4
	Tonic	Nervous system	DMBU	4
	Antiseptic, immunostimulant	Infectious diseases, viral diseases	DMU	4
	Immunostimulant	Leukocyte formation stimulant	DMU	5
	Stimulant, tonic, uplifting	Anemia, asthenia, convalescence	DMB	4
	Blood fluidifier, hypotensive,	Hypertension, hyperviscosity	MBU	4
	Antivirus	Herpes, immune system (low)	DMB	3
	Drainer, lymphatic stimulant	Cellulitis, obesity, water retention	MBCU	4
	Mind, emotion, psyche			
	Antidepressant, uplifting	Anxiety, depression	DMB	4
Lemongrass (*Cymbopogon citratus/* Graminae)	Body and skin care			
	Astringent, tonic	Open pores	FCLO	3
	Medicinal			
	Deodorant, deodorizer, disinfectant	Sanitation	D	3
	Insect repellent	Mosquitos	DLU	2
	Stimulant	Digestive problems	MBC	3
	Digestive, stomachic	Digestive problems	MBC	3
	Regulator	Parasympathic system	DMB	3
	Antiseptic	Infectious diseases	DMBCU	3
	Contraindications			
	Irritant (skin)	Neat or in high concentration	MBFCLOU	2

Essential Oils Reference Table (continued)

Plant name (*Genus species/* family)	Property	Indication	Use	Power
Lime (*Citrus limetta/* Rutaceae)	Medicinal			
	Refreshing	Hot climates	DMBLU	4
	Digestive, stimulant	Digestive problems	MBC	4
	Control of liquid processes	Lymphatic system and secretions, secretions	MBCU	3
	Hepatobiliary stimulant	Gall bladder congestion, liver	MCU	4
	Tonic	Nervous system	DMBU	4
	Stimulant, tonic, uplifting	Anemia, asthenia, convalescence	DMB	3
	Drainer, lymphatic stimulant	Obesity, water retention	MBCU	3
	Antiseptic, antispasmodic	Asthma, bronchitis, catarrhal condition	D	3
	Mind, emotion, psyche			
	Antidepressant, uplifting	Anxiety, depression	DMB	4
Litsea cubeba (Graminae)	Body and skin care			
	Healing, soothing	Dermatitis	MFCLOU	3
	Medicinal			
	Deodorant, deodorizer, disinfectant	Sanitation, epidemics	D	3
	Stimulant	Digestive problems	MBC	3
Lovage root (*Legusticum levisticum/* Umbelliferae)	Medicinal			
	Cleanser, depurative, drainer	Accumulation (toxins, fluids)	MBFCLO	3
	Stimulant, digestive stimulant	Digestive problems, intestines	MBC	3
	Stimulant	Kidneys	MBCU	3
	Revitalizing, stimulant	Anemia, asthenia	DMB	3
	Carminative	Aerophagy, flatulence	MBCU	3
		gout, rheumatism	MBCU	2
	Antispasmodic	Digestive spasms	MBCU	2
	Diuretic	Cystitis, albuminuria	MBCU	4
	Emmenagogue	Amenorrhea, dysmenorrhea	MBCU	3
	Diuretic	Edema, urine retention, water retention	MBCU	3
	Diuretic	Edema, water retention	MBCU	3
Marjoram, wild Spanish (*Thymus mastichina/* Labiatae)	Medicinal			
	Calming	Respiratory system	DMBCU	2
	Antispasmodic	Spasms digestive, spasms respiratory	DMCU	4
	Analgesic, sedative	Migraine	DCU	4
	Analgesic, sedative	Arthritis, rheumatism	MBCU	3

Essential Oils Reference Table (continued)

Plant name (*Genus species/* family)	Property	Indication	Use	Power
	Mind, emotion, psyche			
	Calming, sedative	Insomnia, nervous tension	DMBU	3
Marjoram (*Origanum marjorana* and *marjorana hortensi/* Labiatae)	Medicinal			
	Antispasmodic	Digestive spasms, respiratory spasms	DMBU	4
	Antispasmodic, emmenagogue	Amenorrhea, dysmenorrhea, premenstrual syndrome	MBCU	3
	Hypotensor, vasodilator	Hypertension	MBU	4
	Analgesic, sedative,	Migraine	DCU	4
	Analgesic, sedative	Arthritis, rheumatism	MBCU	3
	Antispasmodic, digestive	Dyspepsia, flatulence	MBCU	2
	Mind, emotion, psyche			
	Appeasing	Astral body	DMBU	4
	Calming, sedative	Insomnia, nervous tension tension	DMBU	4
Melissa (*Melissa officinalis/* Labiatae)	Body and skin care			
	Antiseptic, cytophilactic	Acne, dermatitis, eczema	FCLO	3
	Medicinal			
	Stimulant	Metabolism, vital centers	DMBU	4
	Antivirus	Viral diseases	DMU	4
	Calming, sedative	Insomnia, migraine, nervous tension	DMBC	4
	Mind, emotion, psyche			
	Appeasing	Astral body	DMBU	4
	Antidepressant, calming	Depression, neurasthenia	DMB	5
	Stimulant	Heart chakra	DU	5
	Appeasing, soothing, uplifting	Emotional shock, grief	DMBU	5
Mugwort (*Artemisia vulgaris/* Compositae)	Medicinal			
	Emmenagogue	Amenorrhea, dysmenorrhea, menopause, premenstrual syndrome	MBCU	5
	Analgesic	Teething pain, toothache	U	4
	Balancing	Feminine reproductive system	DMBCU	5
	Cholagogue	Hepatobiliary disorders	MBCU	3
	Vermifuge	Ascaris, oxyurides	MMBU	3
	Mind, emotion, psyche			
	Opening	Dream, psychic work	DU	5
	Contraindications			
	Abortive	Pregnancy	DMBU	4

Essential Oils Reference Table (continued)

Plant name (*Genus species*/family)	Property	Indication	Use	Power
Myrrh (*Commiphora myrrha*/ Burseraceae)	Body and skin care			
	Revitalizing, tonic	Aged skin, wrinkles	FCLO	4
	Medicinal			
	Cooling, drying	Inflammations	FCLU	4
	Regulator	Secretions	MBCU	4
	Balsamic, expectorant	Asthma, catarrhal condition, cough	D	4
	Antiseptic (pulmonary)	Lungs	DUC	3
	Cooling, drying, vulnerary	Infected wounds	FCLOU	4
	Fungicidal	Thrush	Douche	4
	Antiseptic, astringent	Cough, mouth ulcers and inflammations, sore throat	U	4
	Mind, emotion, psyche			
	Fortifying	Mind, psychic centers	DU	5
	Stimulant	Third eye, crown chakra	DU	4
Myrtle (*Myrtus communis*/ Myrtaceae)	Medicinal			
	Balancing, reequilibrating	Energy imbalance	DMB	4
	Antiseptic, stimulant	Respiratory system	DMBCU	5
	Antiseptic	Infectious diseases	DMBCU	4
	Antiseptic (urinary)	Urinary infections	MBC	4
	Balsamic, expectorant	Asthma, bronchitis, tuberculosis	DMBCU	5
Neroli (*Citrus vulgaris*/ Rutaceae)	Body and skin care			
	Soothing	Sensitive skin	FCLO	5
	Medicinal			
	Hypotensor, sedative	Palpitations	DMBC	3
	Mind, emotion, psyche			
	Sedative	Hysteria, insomnia, nervous tension, nervousness	DMBU	5
	Antidepressant, sedative	Emotional shock, grief	DMBU	5
	Stimulant	Heart chakra	DU	5
Niaouli (*Melaleuca viridiflora*/ Myrtaceae)	Medicinal			
	Balancing, reequilibrating	Energy imbalance	DMB	4
	Antiseptic, stimulant	Respiratory system	DMBCU	5
	Antiseptic	Infectious diseases	DMBCU	4
	Antiseptic (urinary)	Urinary infections	MBC	4
	Balsamic, expectorant	Asthma, bronchitis, tuberculosis	DMBCU	5
	Tissue stimulant	Acne, burns, wounds	CLU	4
	Anticatarrhal	Catarrhal condition	D	5
	Antiseptic, expectorant	Sinusitis	DU	5

Essential Oils Reference Table (continued)

Plant name (*Genus species/* family)	Property	Indication	Use	Power
Nutmeg (*Myristica fragrans/* Myristicaceae)	Medicinal			
	Stimulant	Digestive problems	MBC	4
	Analgesic	Pain (muscular and articular), neuralgia, rheumatism	MBCU	3
	Aphrodisiac	Impotence	MBCU	3
	Carminative	Flatulence	MBCU	3
	Antiseptic	Intestines	MBC	3
	Mind, emotion, psyche			
	Stimulant	Nervous and intellectual fatigue	DMB	3
	Contraindications			
	Stupefying, toxic	High doses		3
Orange (*Citrus auranthium/* Rutaceae)	Medicinal			
	Digestive, stimulant	Digestive problems	MBC	3
	Control of liquid processes	Lymphatic system and secretions, secretions	MBCU	2
	Drainer, lymphatic stimulant	Obesity, water retention	MBCU	3
	Hypotensor, sedative	Palpitations	DMBC	2
	Digestive, stimulant	Digestive problems	MBC	3
	Mind, emotion, psyche			
	Sedative	Hysteria, insomnia, nervous tension	DMBU	3
Oregano (*Origanum vulgare/* Labiatae)	Medicinal			
	Stimulant	Metabolism, respiratory system, vital centers	DMBU	4
	Stimulant	Metabolism	DMBU	4
	Stimulant	Respiratory system	DMBCU	4
	Antitoxic, antivirus	Viral diseases	DMU	5
	Antiseptic, cytophilactic	Abscess, burns, wounds	CLU	3
	Antiseptic, antispasmodic	Asthma, bronchitis, catarrhal condition	D	3
	Antiseptic, antitoxic	Infectious diseases	DMBCU	3
	Antiseptic	Blennorrhea, cystitis	MBCU	3
	Revulsive, rubefacient	Circulation, pain (muscular and articular), circulation (capillary)	MBCLOU	4
	Contraindications			
	Irritant (skin)	Neat or in high concentration	FC	4
Palmarosa (*Cymbopogon martini/* Graminae)	Body and skin care			
	Antiseptic, cell regenerator	Acne, dermatitis, skin care	FCLO	3
	Antiseptic, cell regenerator stimulant	Skin care, general skin care	FCLO	3

Essential Oils Reference Table (continued)

Plant name (*Genus species/family*)	Property	Indication	Use	Power
	Moisturizer, soothing	Dry skin	FCLO	3
	Medicinal			
	Stimulant	Digestive problems	MBC	3
Patchouli (*Pogostemon patchouli/* Labiatae)	Body and skin care			
	Antiphlogistic, regenerator	Acne, dermatitis, eczema	FCLO	4
	Tissue regenerator	Aged skin, cracked and chapped skin, wrinkles	FCLO	4
	Fungicidal, tissue regenerator	Impetigo	FCL	3
	Regulator	Seborrhea	FCLO	3
	Decongestant	Skin care	FCLO	3
	Medicinal			
	Fungicidal	Dandruff, fungal infections	CLU	4
	Mind, emotion, psyche			
	Appeasing	Astral body	DMBU	4
	Antidepressant, calming	Anxiety, neurasthenia	DMB	4
Pennyroyal (*Mentha pelugium/* Labiatae)	Medicinal			
	Digestive, stomachic	Dyspepsia, gastralgia, nausea, vomiting	MCU	4
	Emmenagogue	Amenorrhea, dysmenorrhea	MBCU	4
	Insect repellent	Fleas, mosquitos	DLU	4
	Contraindications			
	Abortive	Pregnancy	DMBU	5
	Toxic	Ingestion		3
Pepper (*Piper nigrum/* Piperaceae)	Medicinal			
	Stimulant	Digestive problems, nervous system	DMBU	3
	Aphrodisiac	Impotence	MBCU	3
	Antitoxic	Food poisoning	MU	3
	Digestive, stomachic	Dyspepsia	MCU	3
	Analgesic, rubefacient	Pain (muscular and articular), neuralgia, rheumatism	MBCU	3
	Febrifuge	Fever	MBCU	2
	Mind, emotion, psyche			
	Stimulant	Root chakra	MU	3
	Comforting	Ungroundedness	DMBU	3
Peppermint (*Mentha piperita/* Labiatae)	Body and skin care			
	Cleanser, decongestant	Acne, dermatitis	MFCLOU	4
	Medicinal			
	Stimulant	Metabolism, nervous system,	DMBU	4

Essential Oils Reference Table (continued)

Plant name (*Genus species/family*)	Property	Indication	Use	Power
		respiratory system, vital centers		
	Antiseptic	Infectious diseases	DMBCU	3
	Antiseptic, antispasmodic	Asthma, bronchitis, catarrhal condition	D	3
	Decongestant	Sinusitis	DU	4
	Calming, cephalic	Headache, migraine	DCU	4
	Stimulant (nervous system)	Fainting, vertigo	DC	4
	Digestive, stomachic	Dyspepsia, gastralgia, nausea, vomiting	MCU	5
	Cholagogue, hepatic	Hepatobiliary disorders	MBCU	4
	Febrifuge	Fever	MBCU	4
	Aphrodisiac	Impotence	MBCU	4
	Analgesic, antineuralgic	Pain (muscular and articular), neuralgia,	MBCU	4
	Mind, emotion, psyche			
	Antidepressant, tonic	Depression, neurasthenia	DMB	4
	Stimulant (nervous system)	Fatigue, mental fatigue, mental strain	DMBU	5
Petitgrain biguarade or bitter orange leaves (Rutaceae)	Medicinal			
	Digestive, stimulant	Digestive problems	MBC	3
	Antispasmodic, digestive	Dyspepsia, flatulence	MBCU	3
	Mind, emotion, psyche			
	Clarifying, refreshing	Confusion	DMBU	4
	Antidepressant, uplifting	Anxiety, depression	DMB	3
	Stimulant, tonic	Memory (poor), mental fatigue, mental strain, nervous system	DMBU	4
Pine (*Pinus sylvestris/* Coniferae)	Medicinal			
	Warming	Respiratory weakness	DMBU	3
	Tonic	Glandular system, nervous system, respiratory system	DMBCU	3
	Antiseptic (urinary)	Genitourinary infections, urinary infections	MBC	3
	Expectorant, pectoral	Colds, sore throat	U	4
	Mind, emotion, psyche			
	Appeasing, sedative	Anxiety, stress	DMB	3
Rose (*Rosa centifolia* and *damascena/* Rosaceae)	Body and skin care			
	Cell regenerator	Aged skin, eczema, sensitive skin, wrinkles	FCLO	5
	Moisturizer	Dry skin	FCLO	4

Essential Oils Reference Table (continued)

Plant name (*Genus species/ family*)	Property	Indication	Use	Power
	Medicinal			
	Regulator	Feminine reproductive system	DMBCU	4
	Aphrodisiac	Frigidity, impotence	MBCU	4
	Astringent, hemostatic	Hemorrhage	CLU	3
	Mind, emotion, psyche			
	Stimulant	Heart chakra	DU	5
	Uplifting	Emotional shock, grief	DMBU	5
	Antidepressant, uplifting	Depression, nervous tension, sadness	DMBU	5
Rosemary (*Rosamarinus officinalis/* Labiatae)	Body and skin care			
	Antiseptic, cytophilactic	Acne, dermatitis, eczema	FCLO	4
	Regulator of seborrhea	Dry skin	FCLO	3
	Rejuvenating	Aged skin, wrinkles	FCLO	4
	Regulator, scalp stimulant	Dandruff, hair loss, oily hair	LO	4
	Medicinal			
	Antiseptic, cytophilactic	Abscess, burns, wounds	CLU	3
	Antiseptic, antispasmodic	Asthma, bronchitis, catarrhal condition	D	3
	Stimulant	Adrenocortical glands, metabolism, respiratory system, vital centers	DMBU	4
	Tonic	Anemia, asthenia, debility	DMB	4
	Stimulant (hepatobiliary)	Cholecystitis, cirrhosis, gall bladder congestion, hangover, jaundice	DMBCU	4
	Cardiotonic	Heart	DMBU	3
	Analgesic, rubefacient	Arthritis, pain (muscular and articular)	MCU	3
	Mind, emotion, psyche			
	Appeasing	Astral body	DMBU	4
	Antidepressant, uplifting	Depression, neurasthenia	DMB	4
	Tonic (nervous)	Memory (poor), mental fatigue, mental strain	DMBU	4
Rosewood (*Aniba roseaodora/* Lauraceae)	Body and skin care			
	Antiseptic, cell regenerator	Acne, dermatitis, skin care	FCLO	5
	Cell regenerator, regenerator	Aged skin, sensitive skin, wrinkles	FCLO	5
	Medicinal			
	Calming, cephalic	Headache, nausea	DMCU	4
	Mind, emotion, psyche			
	Antidepressant, uplifting	Anxiety, sadness	DMBU	4

Essential Oils Reference Table (continued)

Plant name (*Genus species/family*)	Property	Indication	Use	Power
Sage lavandulifolia (*Salvia officinalis/* Labiatae)	Body and skin care			
	Depurative, healing	Acne, dermatitis, eczema	FCLO	4
	Regulator of seborrhea	Dandruff, hair loss	LO	4
	Medicinal			
	Stimulant	Adrenocortical glands, metabolism, nervous system, vital centers	DMBU	4
	Stimulant	Metabolism	DMBU	4
	Stimulant	Nervous system	DMBU	4
	Stimulant	Adrenocortical glands	MB	4
	Tonic	Anemia, asthenia, debility	DMB	4
	Stimulant (hepatobiliary)	Cholecystitis, jaundice	DMBCU	4
	Hypertensor	Hypotension	DMCU	4
	Emmenagogue	Amenorrhea, dysmenorrhea, menopause, sterility	MBCU	4
	Antisudorific	Sweating (excessive)	MBCLU	4
	Mind, emotion, psyche			
	Antidepressant, uplifting	Depression, neurasthenia	DMB	4
	Tonic (nervous)	Fatigue, mental fatigue, mental strain	DMBU	4
	Contraindications			
	Abortive, toxic	High doses		4
Sandalwood, Mysore (*Santalum album/* Santalaceae)	Body and skin care			
	Healing, moisturizer, soothing	Acne, cracked and chapped skin, dry skin	FCLO	3
	Medicinal			
	Antiseptic (urinary)	Blennorrhea, cystitis, gonorrhea	LU	3
	Mind, emotion, psyche			
	Elevating, grounding, opening	Third eye, crown chakra	DU	4
	Elevating, grounding, opening	Yoga, meditation, rituals	DU	5
	Antidepressant, euphoric	Depression	DMB	3
Savory (*Satureia montana/* Labiatae)	Medicinal			
	Stimulant	Nervous system	DMBU	4
	Antibiotic, antiseptic	Infectious diseases	DMBCU	5
	Tonic	Anemia, asthenia, debility	DMB	4
	Analgesic, rubefacient	Arthritis, rheumatism	MBCU	4
	Contraindications			
	Irritant (skin)	Neat or in high concentration	BFC	4

Essential Oils Reference Table (continued)

Plant name (*Genus species/ family*)	Property	Indication	Use	Power
Spearmint (*Mentha viridis/* Labiatae)	Body and skin care			
	Cleanser, decongestant	Acne, dermatitis	MFCLOU	3
	Medicinal			
	Decongestant	Sinusitis	DU	3
	Stimulant	Metabolism, nervous system, respiratory system, vital centers	DMBU	3
	Antiseptic, antispasmodic	Asthma, bronchitis, catarrhal condition	D	3
	Calming, cephalic	Headache, migraine	DCU	3
	Digestive, stomachic	Dyspepsia, nausea, vomiting	MCU	4
	Digestive, stomachic	Dyspepsia, gastralgia	MCU	4
	Cholagogue, hepatic	Hepatobiliary disorders	MBCU	4
	Febrifuge	Fever	MBCU	2
	Mind, emotion, psyche			
	Antidepressant, tonic	Depression, neurasthenia	DMB	4
	Stimulant (nervous system)	Fatigue, mental fatigue, mental strain	DMBU	3
Spike (*Lavandula spica/* Labiatae)	Medicinal			
	Stimulant	Respiratory system	DMBCU	3
	Insect repellent	Fleas	DU	4
	Analgesic, rubefacient	Pain (muscular and articular), sport preparation	MCU	4
	Antiseptic, cytophilactic	Abscess, burns, wounds	CLU	3
Spruce (*Picea mariana/* Coniferae)	Medicinal			
	Tonic	Glandular system, nervous system, respiratory system	DMBCU	3
	Warming	Respiratory weakness	DMBU	5
	Antiseptic, expectorant	Asthma, bronchitis	DMBC	4
	Mind, emotion, psyche			
	Elevating, grounding, opening	Psychic work	DU	5
	Elevating, grounding, opening	Third eye, crown chakra	DU	5
	Appeasing, sedative	Anxiety, stress	DMB	5
	Elevating, grounding, opening	Yoga, meditation, rituals	DU	5
Tangerine (*Citrus reticulata/* Rutaceae)	Medicinal			
	Digestive, stimulant	Digestive problems	MBC	3
	Control of liquid processes	Lymphatic system and secretions, secretions	MBCU	2

Essential Oils Reference Table (continued)

Plant name (*Genus species/* family)	Property	Indication	Use	Power
	Antispasmodic, digestive	Dyspepsia, flatulence	MBCU	3
	Drainer, lymphatic stimulant	Obesity, water retention	MBCU	2
	Mind, emotion, psyche			
	Sedative	Hysteria, insomnia, nervous tension, nervousness	DMBU	3
	Sedative, soothing	Emotional shock, grief	DMBU	2
Tarragon (*Artemisia dracunculus/* Compositae)	Medicinal			
	Antispasmodic, digestive	Digestive and intestinal spasms, dyspepsia, hiccup	MCU	4
	Carminative	Aerophagia, fermentation	MBC	4
	Vermifuge	Ascarides, oxyurids	MBCU	3
Tea tree (*Melaleuca alternifolia/* Myrtaceae)	Body and skin care			
	Cicatrizant, fungicidal, vulnerary	Abscess, acne, herpes, pruritis, skin irritation, skin rashes	FCLOU	4
	Fungicidal	Dandruff, hair care	LO	4
	Medicinal			
	Antiseptic, stimulant	Respiratory system	DMBCU	5
	Antiinfectious	Infectious diseases	DMBCU	4
	Antiseptic (urinary)	Urinary infections	MBC	4
	Balsamic, expectorant	Asthma, bronchitis, tuberculosis	DMBCU	5
	Fungicidal	Athlete's foot, *Candida,* fungal infections, ringworm, vaginitis	CLOU	5
	Antiinfectious	Infected wounds, sores	CLOU	4
Therebentine (*Pinus maritimus/* Coniferae)	Medicinal			
	Tonic	Glandular system, respiratory system	DMBCU	3
	Antiseptic (urinary)	Genitourinary infections, urinary infections	MBC	4
	Antiseptic, expectorant	Asthma, bronchitis	DMBC	4
	Expectorant, pectoral	Colds, sore throat	U	4
	Antiseptic, expectorant	Asthma, bronchitis	DMBC	4
Thyme, citriodora (*Thymus vulgaris* chem. *citriodora/* Labiatae)	Medicinal			
	Stimulant	Metabolism, nervous system, vital centers	DMBU	4
	Antibiotic, antiseptic	Infectious diseases	DMBCU	3
	Antiseptic, cytophilactic	Abscess, burns, wounds	CLU	3

Essential Oils Reference Table (continued)

Plant name (*Genus species/* family)	Property	Indication	Use	Power
	Antiseptic, antispasmodic	Asthma, bronchitis, catarrhal condition	D	3
	Tonic	Anemia, asthenia, debility	DMB	3
	Mind, emotion, psyche			
	Appeasing	Astral body	DMBU	4
	Antidepressant, uplifting	Depression, neurasthenia	DMB	4
Thyme, lemon (*Thymus hiemalis/* Labiatae)	Body and skin care			
	Healing, soothing	Acne, dermatitis, eczema	FCLO	4
	Medicinal			
	Stimulant	Metabolism, vital centers	DMBU	4
	Antibiotic, antiseptic	Infectious diseases	DMBCU	3
	Antiseptic, cytophilactic	Abscess, burns, wounds	CLU	3
	Calming	Insomnia, palpitations	DMBC	3
	Mind, emotion, psyche			
	Antidepressant, uplifting	Depression, neurasthenia	DMB	3
Thyme, red (*Tymus zygis/* Labiatae)	Medicinal			
	Stimulant	Metabolism, vital centers	DMBU	4
	Antibiotic, antiseptic	Infectious diseases	DMBCU	5
	Antiseptic (intestinal)	Intestinal infections	MCU	5
	Antiseptic (urinary)	Blennorrhea, cystitis	MBCU	3
	Tonic	Anemia, asthenia, debility	DMB	3
	Analgesic, rubefacient	Arthritis, circulation (capillary), rheumatism, sport preparation	MCU	4
	Stimulant circulation capillary	Cellulitis, circulation, obesity	MBCLOU	3
	Stimulant, uplifting	Depression, neurasthenia	DMB	3
	Contraindications			
	Irritant (skin)	Neat or in high concentration	BFC	4
Verbena, lemon (*Lippia citriodora/* Verbenaceae)	Medicinal			
	Hepatobiliary stimulant	Liver	MCU	3
	Calming	Tachycardia	DMBCU	3
	Mind, emotion, psyche			
	Regulator	Neurovegetative system	DMBU	3
	Calming	Nervousness	DMBU	3
Vetiver (*Andropogon muricatus/* Graminae)	Medicinal			
	Rubefacient	Arthritis	MBCU	4
	Mind, emotion, psyche			
	Stimulant	Root chakra	MU	4
	Comforting	Ungroundedness	DMBU	4

Essential Oils Reference Table (continued)

Plant name (*Genus species*/family)	Property	Indication	Use	Power
Ylang-ylang (*Unona odorantissimum*/Anonaceae)	Body and skin care			
	Antiseborrheic	Oily skin	FCLO	3
	Scalp stimulant	Hair growth	LO	3
	Medicinal			
	Hypotensive	Hyperpnea, hypertension, palpitations, tachycardia	DMBCU	4
	Aphrodisiac	Frigidity, impotence	MBCU	4
	Mind, emotion, psyche			
	Antidepressant, euphoric	Depression, menopause, stress	DMB	3
	Sedative	Insomnia, nervous tension	DMBU	3
	Stimulant	Sexual chakra	DMBU	3
	Calming, euphoric	Anger, fear, frustration	DMBU	3

APPENDIX II

Aromatherapy
Therapeutic Index

BEAUTY, SKIN, AND HAIR CARE

Acne
Bergamot, blue chamomile, German chamomile, everlasting, geranium, juniper, lavender, melissa, niaouli, palmarosa, patchouli, peppermint, rosemary, rosewood, sage lavandulifolia, Mysore sandalwood, spearmint, tea tree, lemon thyme.

Application methods: Compress, facial, mask, lotion, face oil/body oil.

Aged Skin
Carrot seed, clary sage, frankincense, geranium, myrrh, patchouli, rose, rosemary, rosewood.

Application methods: Compress, facial, mask, lotion, face oil/body oil, body wrap.

Cracked and Chapped Skin
Benzoin resinoid, patchouli, Mysore sandalwood.

Application methods: Compress, facial, mask, lotion, friction/unguent.

Dandruff
Cedarwood, patchouli, rosemary, sage lavandulifolia, tea tree.

Application methods: Lotion, hair oil, shampoo.

Dermatitis
Benzoin resinoid, blue chamomile, German chamomile, carrot seed, cedarwood, everlasting, geranium, jasmine enfleurage, juniper, lavender, *Litsea cubeba*, melissa, palmarosa, patchouli, peppermint, rosemary, rosewood, sage lavandulifolia, spearmint, lemon thyme.

Application methods: Compress, facial, mask, lotion, massage, face oil/body oil, friction/unguent.

Dry Skin
Clary sage, jasmine enfleurage, palmarosa, rose, rosemary, Mysore sandalwood.

Application methods: Compress, facial, mask, lotion, face oil/body oil.

Eczema
Bergamot, blue chamomile, German chamomile, cedarwood, juniper, lavender, melissa, patchouli, rose, rosemary, sage lavandulifolia, lemon thyme.

Application methods: Compress, facial, mask, lotion, face oil/body oil.

Hair Growth
Bay, clary sage, ylang-ylang.
Application methods: Lotion, face oil/body oil, shampoo.

Hair Loss
Cedarwood, rosemary, sage lavandulifolia, ylang-ylang.
Application methods: Lotion, face oil/body oil, shampoo.

Inflamed Skin
Blue chamomile, German chamomile, clary sage, everlasting.
Application methods: Compress, facial, mask, lotion, face oil/body oil, body wrap.

Oily Hair
Cedarwood, clary sage, rosemary.
Application methods: Lotion, face oil/body oil, shampoo.

Oily Skin
Clary sage, geranium, lavender, lemon, ylang-ylang.
Application methods: Compress, facial, mask, lotion, face oil/body oil.

Seborrhea
Bergamot, patchouli, sage.
Application methods: Compress, facial, mask, lotion, face oil/body oil, body wrap.

Sensitive Skin
Blue chamomile, chamomile mixta, Roman chamomile, German chamomile, everlasting, jasmine enfleurage, neroli, rose, rosewood.
Application methods: Compress, facial, mask, lotion, face oil/body oil, body wrap.

Skin Care
Blue chamomile, German chamomile, everlasting, geranium, lemon, palmarosa, patchouli, rosewood.

Application methods: Compress, facial, mask, lotion, face oil/body oil, body wrap.

Skin Irritation, Skin Rashes
Benzoin resinoid, carrot seed, everlasting, tea tree.
Application methods: Compress, facial, mask, lotion, face oil/body oil, friction/unguent.

Wrinkles
Carrot seed, clary sage, frankincense, myrrh, patchouli, rose, rosemary, rosewood, spikenard.
Application methods: Compress, facial, mask, lotion, face oil/body oil.

MEDICINAL INDICATIONS

Abscess
Blue chamomile, Roman chamomile, German chamomile, everlasting, lavender, oregano, rosemary, spike, tea tree, citriodora, lemon thyme.
Application methods: Compress, facial, mask, lotion, face oil/body oil.

Accumulation (Toxins, Fluids)
Angelica root, birch, caraway seeds, carrot seed, coriander seeds, cumin seeds, fennel, juniper, lovage root.
Application methods: Bath, compress, facials, mask, lotion, massage, face oil/body oil, body wrap.

Adrenocortical Glands
Geranium, rosemary, sage lavandulifolia.
Application methods: Bath, massage.

Aerophagy
Angelica root, aniseed, caraway seeds, cardamom, coriander seeds, cumin seeds, fennel, ginger root, lovage root, tarragon.
Application methods: Bath, compress, massage.

Amenorrhea, Dysmenorrhea

Chamomile mixta, Roman chamomile, German chamomile, carrot seed, clary sage, fennel, lavender, lovage root, marjoram, mugwort, pennyroyal, sage lavandulifolia.

Application methods: Bath, compress, massage, friction/unguent, douche.

Anemia, Asthenia

Angelica root, Roman chamomile, German chamomile, carrot seed, cinnamon bark, clove buds, coriander seeds, cumin seeds, fennel, lemon, lime, lovage root, petitgrain biguarade, rosemary, sage lavandulifolia, savory, thyme citriodora, red thyme.

Application methods: Bath, diffuser, massage.

Anorexia

Angelica root, carrot seed, coriander seeds.

Application methods: Bath, diffuser, massage.

Arthritis

Birch, blue chamomile, Roman chamomile, German chamomile, ginger root, juniper, marjoram, wild Spanish marjoram, rosemary, savory, red thyme, vetiver.

Application methods: Bath, compress, massage, friction/unguent, body wrap.

Asthma

Cajeput, cypress, *Eucalyptus australiana*, *Eucalyptus globulus*, fir, frankincense, hyssop, lavender, lime, myrrh, myrtle, niaouli, oregano, peppermint, rosemary, spearmint, spruce, tea tree, therebentine, thyme citriodora.

Application methods: Bath, compress, diffuser, massage, friction/unguent.

Blennorrhea

Lavender, oregano, Mysore sandalwood, red thyme.

Application methods: Bath, massage, friction/unguent.

Boils

Chamomile (blue, Roman, German), everlasting.

Application methods: Compress, facials, mask, lotion, face oil/body oil.

Bronchitis

Benzoin resinoid, lime, myrtle, niaouli, oregano, peppermint, rosemary, spearmint, spruce, tea tree, therebentine, thyme citriodora.

Application methods: Bath, compress, diffuser, massage.

Bruises

Blue chamomile, geranium, lavender, everlasting.

Application methods: Compress, lotion, friction/unguent.

Burns

Geranium, lavender, lavandin, niaouli, oregano, rosemary, spike, thyme citriodora, lemon thyme.

Application methods: Compress, lotion, friction/unguent.

Candida

Tea tree.

Application methods: Compress, lotion, face oil/body oil, friction/unguent, douche.

Catarrhal Condition

Frankincense, hyssop, lavender, lime, myrrh, niaouli, oregano, peppermint, rosemary, spearmint, thyme citriodora.

Application methods: Diffuser.

Cellulitis

Angelica root, birch, cypress, fennel, geranium, grapefruit, lemon, red thyme.

Application methods: Bath, compress, massage, friction/unguent, body wrap.

Circulation

Cinnamon bark, cinnamon leaf, cypress, lemon, oregano, red thyme.

Application methods: Bath, compress, massage, friction/unguent, body wrap.

Circulation (Capillary)

Oregano, red thyme.

Application methods: Bath, compress, lotion, massage, face oil/body oil, friction/unguent, body wrap.

Colds

Eucalyptus globulus, lavender, pine, spruce, therebentine.

Application methods: Compress, diffuser, massage, friction/unguent.

Convalescence

Angelica root, carrot seed, coriander seeds, cumin seeds, lemon, lime, petitgrain biguarade.

Application methods: Bath, diffuser, massage.

Cough

Benzoin resinoid, cypress, frankincense, myrrh.

Application methods: Diffuser.

Cystitis

Birch, cajeput, cedarwood, juniper, lavender, lovage root, oregano, Mysore sandalwood, red thyme.

Application methods: Bath, compress, massage, friction/unguent.

Debility

Rosemary, sage lavandulifolia, savory, thyme citriodora, red thyme.

Application methods: Bath, diffuser, massage.

Diabetes

Eucalyptus australiana, E. globulus, geranium, juniper.

Application methods: Bath, massage.

Digestive Problems

Angelica root, aniseed, bergamot, Roman chamomile, German chamomile, caraway seeds, cardamom, cinnamon bark, coriander seeds, cumin seeds, fennel, ginger root, grapefruit, lemon, lemongrass, lime, *Litsea cubeba,* lovage root.

Application methods: Bath, compress, massage.

Dyspepsia

Basil, caraway seeds, clove buds, ginger root, hyssop, pennyroyal (*use internally only with guidance of primary care practitioner*), pepper, peppermint, petitgrain biguarade, spearmint, tangerine, tarragon.

Application methods: Compress, massage, friction/unguent.

Energy Deficiency

Caraway seeds, clove buds, cypress.

Application methods: Bath, diffuser, massage.

Energy Imbalance

Benzoin resinoid, cajeput, *Eucalyptus australiana, E. globulus,* myrtle, niaouli.

Application methods: Bath, diffuser, massage.

Fainting

Peppermint.

Application methods: Compress, diffuser.

Feminine Reproductive System

Chamomile (Roman, German), clary sage, fennel, mugwort, rose.

Application methods: Bath, compress, diffuser, massage, friction/unguent, douche.

Fermentations

Caraway seeds, clove buds, tarragon.

Application methods: Bath, compress, massage.

Fever

Ginger root, peppermint.
Application methods: Bath, compress, massage, friction/unguent.

Flatulence

Cardamom, coriander seeds, cumin seeds, fennel, ginger root, lovage root, nutmeg, petitgrain biguarade, tangerine.
Application methods: Bath, compress, massage, friction/unguent.

Fleas

Lavender, lavandin, pennyroyal, spike.
Application methods: Diffuser, friction/unguent.

Frigidity

Clary sage, jasmine enfleurage, rose, ylang-ylang.
Application methods: Bath, compress, diffuser, massage, friction/unguent.

Fungal Infections

Cedarwood, patchouli, tea tree.
Application methods: Compress, lotion, friction/unguent, douche.

Gallbladder Congestion

Lemon, lime, rosemary.
Application methods: Bath, compress, massage, friction/unguent.

Gastric Spasms

Basil, ginger root, tarragon.
Application methods: Compress, massage, friction/unguent.

Genitourinary Infections

Fir, juniper, pine, therebentine.
Application methods: Bath, compress, lotion, massage.

Glandular System

Carrot seed, cedarwood, coriander seeds, fennel, fir, juniper, pine, spruce, therebentine.
Application methods: Bath, massage, friction/unguent.

Gout

Angelica root, coriander seeds.
Application methods: Compress, massage, friction/unguent.

Headache

Chamomile mixta, chamomile (Roman, German), lavender, peppermint, rosewood, spearmint.
Application methods: Bath, compress, diffuser, massage, friction/unguent.

Hemorrhage

Everlasting, geranium, rose.
Application methods: Compress, lotion, friction/unguent.

Hemorrhoids

Cypress.
Application methods: Compress, lotion, friction/unguent.

Hepatobiliary Disorders

Carrot seed, mugwort, pennyroyal, peppermint, spearmint.
Application methods: Bath, compress, massage, friction/unguent.

Herpes

Lemon, tea tree.
Application methods: Compress, face oil/body oil, friction/unguent.

Hiccup

Tarragon.
Application methods: Compress, massage, friction/unguent.

Hypertension

Lemon, marjoram, ylang-ylang.
Application methods: Bath, massage, friction/unguent.

Hypotension

Hyssop, sage lavandulifolia.
Application methods: Compress, diffuser, massage, friction/unguent.

Immune System (Low)

Lemon, tea tree.
Application methods: Bath, diffuser, massage.

Impotence

Cardamom, champaca flowers, clary sage, clove buds, ginger root, jasmine enfleurage, nutmeg, pepper, peppermint, rose, Mysore sandalwood, ylang-ylang.
Application methods: Bath, compress, massage, friction/unguent.

Infectious Diseases

Bay, cajeput, cinnamon bark, cinnamon leaf, citronella, clove buds, *Eucalyptus australiana, E. citriodora, E. globulus,* geranium, lavender, lavandin, lemon, lemongrass, *Litsea cubeba,* myrtle, niaouli, oregano, peppermint, savory, tea tree, red thyme.
Application methods: Bath, compress, diffuser, massage, friction/unguent.

Inflamed Joint

Chamomile (blue, German, Roman).
Application methods: Bath, compress, friction/unguent.

Inflammations

Frankincense, myrrh.
Application methods: Compress, facials, mask, lotion, friction/unguent.

Insomnia

Chamomile mixta, chamomile (German, Roman), cistus, lavender, marjoram, wild Spanish marjoram, melissa, neroli, orange, spikenard, tangerine, lemon thyme, ylang-ylang.
Application methods: Bath, diffuser, massage, friction/unguent.

Insufficient Milk (Nursing)

Fennel.
Application methods: Compress, massage, friction/unguent.

Intestinal Infections

Basil, bergamot, cinnamon (bark, leaf), red thyme.
Application methods: Compress, massage, friction/unguent.

Intestines

Lovage root, nutmeg.
Application methods: Bath, compress, massage.

Kidneys

Birch, geranium, lovage root.
Application methods: Bath, compress, massage, friction/unguent.

Liver

Chamomile mixta, chamomile (blue, German, Roman), everlasting.
Application methods: Compress, massage, friction/unguent.

Liver and Spleen Congestion

Chamomile (German, Roman), everlasting, lemon, lemon verbena, lime.
Application methods: Compress, massage, friction/unguent.

Lymphatic System and Secretions
Grapefruit, lemon, lime.
Application methods: Bath, massage, friction/unguent.

Menopause
Chamomile mixta, chamomile (German, Roman), geranium, jasmine enfleurage, lavender, mugwort, sage lavandulifolia, ylang-ylang.
Application methods: Bath, compress, diffuser, massage, friction/unguent.

Metabolism
Lavender, melissa, oregano, peppermint, rosemary, sage lavandulifolia, spearmint, thyme citriodora, lemon thyme, red thyme.
Application methods: Bath, diffuser, massage, friction/unguent.

Migraine
Angelica root, aniseed, basil, chamomile mixta, chamomile (German, Roman), caraway seeds, coriander seeds, cumin seeds, ginger root, lavender, marjoram, wild Spanish marjoram, melissa, peppermint, spearmint.
Application methods: Compress, diffuser, friction/unguent.

Mosquitos
Citronella, geranium, lavandin, pennyroyal.
Application methods: Diffuser, lotion, friction/unguent.

Moths
Lavender, lavandin.
Application methods: Diffuser, friction/unguent.

Nausea
Peppermint, rosewood, spearmint.
Application methods: Compress, diffuser, massage, friction/unguent.

Neuraliga
Bay, clove buds, nutmeg, pepper, peppermint.
Application methods: Bath, compress, massage, friction/unguent.

Obesity
Angelica root, birch, fennel, grapefruit, lemon, lime, orange, red thyme.
Application methods: Bath, compress, massage, friction/unguent, body wrap.

Pain (Muscular and Articular)
Bay, birch, clove buds, nutmeg, oregano, pepper, peppermint, rosemary, spike.
Application methods: Bath, compress, massage, friction/unguent.

Palpitations
Lavender, melissa, neroli, lemon thyme, spikenard, ylang-ylang.
Application methods: Bath, compress, diffuser, massage.

Perspiration (Especially Feet)
Cypress, sage.
Application methods: Bath, compress, lotion, massage, friction/unguent.

Premenstrual Syndrome
Carrot seed, clary sage, fennel, lavender, marjoram, mugwort.
Application methods: Bath, compress, massage, friction/unguent, douche.

Respiratory System
Bay, cajeput, cedarwood, clove buds, cypress, *Eucalyptus australian, E. globulus,* fir, hyssop, lavender, lavandin, myrtle, niaouli, oregano, peppermint, pine, rosemary, spearmint, spike, spruce, tea tree, therebentine.
Application methods: Bath, compress, diffuser, massage, friction/unguent.

Respiratory Weakness
Fir, pine, spruce.
Application methods: Bath, diffuser, massage, friction/unguent.

Rheumatism
Birch, cajeput, coriander seeds, ginger root, juniper, marjoram, wild Spanish marjoram, nutmeg, pepper, rosemary, savory, red thyme.
Application methods: Bath, compress, massage, friction/unguent.

Sanitation
Citronella, *Eucalyptus citriodora*, lavandin, lemongrass, litsea cubeda.
Application methods: Diffuser.

Secretions
Benzoin resinoid, elemi, frankincense, grapefruit, lemon, lime, myrrh.
Application methods: Bath, compress, massage, friction/unguent.

Sinusitis
Cajeput, *Eucalyptus australiana, E. globulus,* lavender, myrtle, niaouli, peppermint, spearmint.
Application methods: Diffuser, friction/unguent.

Sore Throat
Geranium, ginger root, myrrh, pine, spruce, therebentine.
Application methods: Friction/unguent, gargle.

Spasms, Digestive
Angelica root, aniseed, caraway seeds, coriander seeds, cumin seeds, fennel, marjoram, wild Spanish marjoram.
Application methods: Bath, compress, massage, friction/unguent.

Tachycardia
Lemon verbena, spikenard, ylang-ylang.
Application methods: Bath, compress, diffuser, massage, friction/unguent.

Teething Pain
Chamomile (blue, German, Roman), mugwort.
Application methods: Friction/unguent, gargle.

Tonsillitis
Blue chamomile, geranium, ginger root.
Application methods: Friction/unguent, gargle.

Toothache
Chamomile, (blue, German, Roman), clove buds, mugwort.
Application methods: Friction/unguent, gargle.

Tuberculosis
Cajeput, *Eucalyptus australiana, E. globulus,* myrtle, niaouli, tea tree.
Application methods: Bath, compress, diffuser, massage, friction/unguent.

Urinary Infections
Cajeput, cedarwood, cistus, clove buds, *Eucalyptus australiana, E. globulus,* fir, juniper, myrtle, niaouli, pine, tea tree, therebentine.
Application methods: Bath, compress, massage.

Varicosis
Cypress, lemon.
Application methods: Compress, lotion, friction/unguent.

Viral Diseases
Lemon, melissa, oregano.
Application methods: Diffuser, massage, friction/unguent.

Vital Centers

Basil, ginger root, hyssop, lavender, melissa, oregano, peppermint, rosemary, sage lavandulifolia, spearmint, thyme citriodora, lemon thyme, red thyme.

Application methods: Bath, diffuser, massage, friction/unguent.

Vomiting

Peppermint, spearmint.

Application methods: Compress, massage, friction/unguent.

Water Retention

Angelica root, birch, cypress, fennel, grapefruit, lemon, lime, lovage root, orange.

Application methods: Bath, compress, massage, friction/unguent, body wrap.

Whooping Cough

Cypress, hyssop.

Application methods: Compress, diffuser, massage.

Wounds

Benzoin resinoid, everlasting, geranium, lavender, lavandin, niaouli, oregano, rosemary, spike, thyme citriodora, lemon thyme.

Application methods: Compress, lotion, friction/unguent.

Wounds (Infected)

Caraway seeds, clove buds, elemi, frankincense, myrrh, tea tree.

Application methods: Compress, facials, lotion, face oil/body oil, friction/unguent.

MIND, EMOTIONS, AND PSYCHE

Anger

Chamomile (German, Roman), ylang-ylang.

Application methods: Bath, diffuser, massage, friction/unguent.

Anxiety

Benzoin resinoid, bergamot, cedarwood, fir, jasmine enfleurage, lemon, lime, patchouli, petitgrain biguarade, pine, rosewood, spikenard, spruce.

Application methods: Bath, diffuser, massage, friction/unguent.

Astral Body

Lavender, lavandin, marjoram, melissa, patchouli, rosemary, thyme citriodora.

Application methods: Bath, diffuser, massage, friction/unguent.

Confidence (Lack of)

Jasmine enfleurage.

Application methods: Bath, diffuser, massage, friction/unguent.

Confusion

Petitgrain biguarade.

Application methods: Bath, diffuser, massage, friction/unguent.

Depression

Bargamot, clary sage, geranium, jasmine enfleurage, lavender, lemon, lime, melissa, peppermint, petitgrain biguarade, rose, rosemary, sage lavandulifolia, Mysore sandalwood, spearmint, thyme citriodora, lemon thyme, red thyme, ylang-ylang.

Application methods: Bath, diffuser, massage.

Depression (Postnatal)

Clary sage, jasmine enfleurage.

Application methods: Bath, diffuser, massage.

Dream

Mugwort, clary sage.

Application methods: Diffuser, friction/unguent.

Emotional Shock

Melissa, neroli, rose.

Application methods: Bath, diffuser, massage, friction/unguent.

Fatigue, Nervous, Intellectual

Basil, clove buds, juniper, nutmeg.

Application methods: Bath, diffuser, massage.

Grief

Melissa, neroli, rose.

Application methods: Bath, diffuser, massage, friction/unguent.

Hysteria

Neroli, orange, tangerine.

Application methods: Bath, diffuser, massage.

Memory (Poor)

Basil, clove buds, ginger root, juniper, petitgrain biguarade, rosemary.

Application methods: Bath, diffuser, massage, friction/unguent.

Mental Fatigue, Mental Strain

Basil, caraway seeds, ginger root, peppermint, petitgrain biguarade, rosemary, sage lavandulifolia, spearmint.

Application methods: Bath, diffuser, massage, friction/unguent.

Mind

Frankincense, myrrh.

Application methods: Bath, diffuser, massage, friction/unguent.

Nervous System

Bergamot, cedarwood, cinnamon bark, cumin seeds, fir, lemon, lime, pepper, peppermint, petitgrain biguarade, pine, sage lavandulifolia, savory, spearmint, spruce, thyme citriodora.

Application methods: Bath, diffuser, massage, friction/unguent.

Nervous Tension

Geranium, lavender, marjoram, wild Spanish marjoram, melissa, neroli, orange, rose, tangerine, ylang-ylang.

Application methods: Bath, diffuser, massage, friction/unguent.

Nervousness

Cistus, neroli, orange, tangerine, lemon verbena.

Application methods: Bath, diffuser, massage, friction/unguent.

Neurasthenia

Lavender, melissa, patchouli, peppermint, rosemary, sage lavandulifolia, spearmint, thyme citriodora, lemon thyme, red thyme.

Application methods: Bath, diffuser, massage.

Neurovegetative System

Basil, ginger root, lemon verbena.

Application methods: Bath, diffuser, massage, friction/unguent.

Psychic Centers

Cistus, elemi, frankincense, myrrh.

Application methods: Diffuser, friction/unguent.

Psychic Work

Cedarwood, cistus, mugwort, spruce.

Application methods: Diffuser, friction/unguent.

Sadness

Benzoin resinoid, jasmine enfleurage, rose, rosewood.

Application methods: Bath, diffuser, massage, friction/unguent.

Stress

Cedarwood, fir, pine, spruce, ylang-ylang.
Application methods: Bath, diffuser, massage.

Tantrum

Chamomile (German, Roman).
Application methods: Bath, diffuser, massage, friction/unguent.

Ungroundedness

Pepper, vetiver.
Application methods: Bath, diffuser, massage, friction/unguent.

Yoga, Meditation, Rituals

Cedarwood, cistus, Mysore sandalwood, spruce.
Application methods: Diffuser, friction/unguent.

CHAKRAS AND ENERGY CENTERS

Crown Chakra

Benzoin resinoid cistus, frankincense, myrrh, Mysore sandalwood, spruce.
Application methods: Diffuser, friction/unguent.

Heart Chakra

Benzoin resinoid, melissa, neroli, rose.
Application methods: Diffuser, friction/unguent.

Root Chakra

Pepper, spikenard, vetiver.
Application methods: Massage, friction/unguent.

Sexual Chakra

Champaca flowers, jasmine enfleurage, ylang-ylang.
Application methods: Bath, diffuser, massage, friction/unguent.

Third Eye

Cistus, frankincense, myrrh, Mysore sandalwood, spruce.
Application methods: Diffuser, friction/unguent.

APPENDIX III

Resource Guide

SUPPLIERS

Aroma Véra (Manufacturer)
5901 Rodeo Rd.
Los Angeles, CA 90016-4312
(800) 669-9514, (310) 280-0407;
Fax: (310) 280-0395
Aroma Véra offers a comprehensive line of essential oils and essential oil combinations, mostly of wild or organic origins. Its products cover skin, body, and hair care, environmental fragrancing, and gift sets and accessories, including jewelry. The company's products may be purchased at health food stores, boutiques, and salons throughout the United States and Canada, or directly from the company via mail order. The company also offers education.

Frontier Cooperative Herbs (Manufacturer)
1 Frontier Rd.
Norway, IA 52318
(319) 227-7996
Frontier Cooperative Herbs is one of the largest herb distributors in the United States and also offers a large selection of essential oils. Recently, Frontier Cooperative Herbs acquired Aura Cacia, another prominent aromatherapy supplier. The company's products are sold primarily through health food stores.

Original Swiss Aromatics (Manufacturer)
P.O. Box 606
San Rafael, CA 94915
(415) 479-9120
Original Swiss Aromatics offers a wide choice of essential oils, mostly of wild or organic origins, skin and body care products, and education. The company's products are available through naturopathic doctors and via mail order.

Oshadhi (Importer from Germany)
15 Monarch Bay Plaza, Ste. 346
Monarch Beach, CA 92629
(714) 240-1104
Oshadhi carries a comprehensive range of essential oils, many of wild or organic origins, along with skin care, body care, and fragrancing products. The company's products can be found in health food stores.

Simpler's Botanical Company
  (Manufacturer)
P.O. Box 39
Forestville, CA 95436-0039
Simpler's sells primarily herbs and essential oils. The company also offers a limited supply of skin and body care products. The products are available via mail order and may also be found in a few stores.

Tisserand Aromatherapy (Importer from United Kingdom)
P.O. Box 750428
Petaluma, CA 94975-0428
(707) 769-5120
The company is named after Robert Tisserand, the author of several popular aromatherapy books and a consultant for Tisserand Aromatherapy. The company offers essential oils and skin and body care products, which can be purchased in health food stores and boutiques.

True Essence Aromatherapy (Distributor)
2203 Westmount Rd. NW
Calgary, Alberta T2N 3N5
Canada
(403) 283-5653
In Canada only: (800) 563-8938
True Essence Aromatherapy carries a comprehensive range of essential oils, body care, skin care, and fragrancing products, available by mail order in Canada. It also houses a skin care and body care clinic on the premises.

La Marquise–Texas (Distributor)
2323 Center St.
Deer Park, TX 77536
(713) 930-8126 and (800) 633-7498
La Marquise–Texas carries a comprehensive range of essential oils, body care, skin care, and fragrancing products.

The Vitamin Shoppe
4700 Westside Ave. North
Bergenfield, NJ 07047
(201) 866-7711

RETAIL STORES

United States

California
The Bey's Garden
2919 Main St.
Santa Monica, CA 90405
(310) 399-5420
The Bey's Garden offers a complete range of aromatherapy products and services. The entire Aroma Véra line is available, along with a blending bar for customizing. The Bey's Garden also provides skin and body care treatments, including massage, facials, and body wraps.

Mother's Market
225 East 17th St.
Costa Mesa, CA 92627
(714) 631-4741
19770 Beach Blvd.
Huntington Beach, CA 92648
(714) 963-6667

Nature's Garden
Hanford Mall, Highway 198
Hanford, CA 93230
(209) 583-1345
Retail only.

The Remedy Store
1590-D Rosecrans Blvd.
Manhattan Beach, CA 90266
(310) 643-9050

Palmetto
1034 Montana Ave.
Santa Monica, CA 90403
(310) 395-6687

Florida
Natural Scents
483 Mandalay Ave.
Clearwater Beach, FL 36430
(813) 447-1704

Maryland
Pampered Body
806 South Boardwalk, Unit 11
Ocean City, MD 21842
(410) 289-1491

Massachusetts
Essentials
Mashpee Commons
Mashpee, MA 02649
(508) 539-2898

Taproot
617 Carpenter Rd.
Whitensville, MA 01588
(508) 234-2301

New York
Body Mind & Soul
191 Walt Whitman Rd.
Huntington Station, NY 11746
(516) 423-8400

Ayurveda Prana Foods
129 1st Ave.
New York, NY 10003
(212) 260-1218

Lemongrass
367 W. Broadway
New York, NY 10013-2209
(212) 343-0900

Tennessee
Squash Blossom and Market
5101 Sanderlin St., Ste. 124
Memphis, TN 38117
(901) 685-2293

Texas
Sabia Botanicals
4101 Guadalupe Place #500
Austin, TX 78751
(512) 323-6198

Herb Market
1002 4th Ave.
Carrollton, TX 75006
(214) 446-9503

The Body Journey
10807 Elmdale St.
Houston, TX 77070
(713) 955-6071

Washington
European Soaps Limited
12300 15th Ave. Northeast
Seattle, WA 98125
(206) 361-9143

Washington, DC
Corso Di Fiori
801 Pennsylvania Avenue NW
Washington, DC 20004
(202) 628-1929

Canada

Alberta
Community Natural Foods
1304 10th Ave. SW
Calgary, Alberta T3C 0J1
(403) 229-2383

Counter Clockwise Emporium
Jasper Marketplace, 627 Patricia St.
Jasper, Alberta T0E 1E0
(403) 852-3152

British Columbia

Escents
Store M31 1020 Park Royal South
West Vancouver, BC V7T 1A1
(604) 926-7720

Manitoba

Tess Body Care
290-25 Forks Market Rd.
Winnipeg, Manitoba, R3C 4S8
(204) 942-5800

Tess Body Care
34-1530 18th St.
Brandon, Manitoba, R7A 5C5
(204) 727-1345

Saskatchewan

Heavenly Scents by Sandra
1230 4th St.
Estevan, Saskatchewan, S4A 0W9
(306) 634-5253

AROMATHERAPY TREATMENT CENTERS

United States

Arizona

Salon Phoenix
101 E. Monroe
Phoenix, AZ 85004
(602) 253-1879
Hair salon with retail.

California

The Face Place
133 La Plaza
Palm Springs, CA 92262
(619) 325-7055

The Bey's Garden
2919 Main St.
Santa Monica, CA 90405
(310) 399-5420

A Place to Relax
1410 Guerneville Road, Suite 11
Santa Rosa, CA 95410
(707) 573-3910
Oriental and European technique massage,
reflexology, and retail.

Preston Wyn Salon
14567 Big Basin Way
Saratoga, CA 95070
(408) 741-5525
Massages and facials and a blending bar for
customizing.

Connecticut

Body Boutique
37 East Main St.
Old Avon Village, CT 06001
(203) 677-1103

Total Image Salon
549 Post Rd.
Darien, CT 06820
(203) 655-2523
Offers facials, manicures, pedicures, and retail.

Florida

Hair Studio 2000
955 West Lancaster Rd.
Orlando, FL 32809
(407) 857-0223
Head and shoulder massages, facials, hand
therapy, pedicures, and skin care.

Florida Institute
2001 W. Sample Road, 1st Floor
Pompano Beach, FL 33064
(954) 975-6400
Beauty school with some public retail.

D. G. Body Therapy & Day Spa
1881 Northeast 26th St., Ste. 20
Wilton Manors, FL 33305
(305) 556-3494
Inhalation treatments and massage therapy
by licensed massage therapists.

Massachusetts

Salon Ekos
118 Newbury St.
Boston, MA
(617) 247-8890
Aromatic hair, skin, and body treatments in
addition to aromatherapy workshops. Staffed
by licensed professional with expertise in all
phases of hair designing, cosmetics, and esthetics. Salon EKOS features custom blending services to enhance the lifestyle of great
looks and natural well-being.

Absolute Scentsations
16 Ken Dr.
Gardiner, MA 01440
(508) 632-9923
Skin care treatments, nail care services, and
aromatherapy classes for groups or individuals.

Minnesota

Simonson's Salon and Day Spa
646 East River Rd.
Anoka, MN 55303.
(612) 427-0761

Christal Center
394 Lake Ave. South
Duluth, MN 55802
(218) 722-2411

New Reflections
12760 Bass Lake Rd.
Maple Grove, MN 55369
(612) 559-3185

The Marsh
15000 Minnetonka Blvd.
Minnetonka, MN 55345
(612) 935-2202

New Jersey

Appearance Center
984 Route 166
Toms River, NJ 08753
(908) 244-1155
Manicures, pedicures, scalp treatments, and
facials.

New York

Kimberly—A Day Spa
637 London Rd.
Latham, NY 12110
(518) 785-5868

Carapan
96 5th Ave. #9L
New York, NY 10011
(212) 633-6220
Full skin and body aromatherapy treatment.

Mulcare Beauty Studio & Spa
194-05 Linden Blvd.
St. Albans, NY 11412
(718) 712-1025
Massage, facials, waxing, and retail.

Ohio

Ten Minute Backrub
18 West 4th St.
Cincinnati, OH 45202
(513) 721-7822
Massage plus retail.

Ten Minute Backrub
11700 Princeton Pike, #B219
Cincinnati, OH 45246
(606) 525-0390
Massage plus retail.

Texas

With Class—A Day Spa
621-B Chase Dr.
Tyler, TX 75701
(903) 581-1745

Vermont

Green Door Spa
Route 7 RR 1 Village Mall
Manchester, VT 05255
(802) 362-1528

Canada

Alberta

Parks Canada Upper Hot Springs Spa
Box 900
Banff, Alberta T01 0C0
(403) 762-1515

Grandin Health and Healing Center
Rivercrest Plaza
367 St. Albert Trail
St. Albert, Alberta T8N 0R1
(403) 459-7796
Offers massage and retail.

British Columbia

Mo's Studio
Unit 17 5901 East Broadway
Burnaby, British Columbia V5B 2X4.
(604) 298-6991

Pure
200-329 North Rd.
Coquitlam, British Columbia V3K 3V8
(604) 936-8288
Massage, reflexology, and retail.

Nova Scotia

The Summit Aesthetic Spa
Park Lane Mall
5657 Spring Garden Rd.
Halifax, Nova Scotia B3J 3R4
(902) 423-3888
Massage, esthetics services, and retail.

Ontario

Country Comforts by Marnie
109 Daniel St. N
Arnprior, Ontario K7S 2L1
(613) 623-9656
Facials, manicures, pedicures, and retail.

AROMATHERAPY EDUCATION CENTERS

Michael Scholes School for Aromatic
  Studies
117 North Robertson Blvd.
Los Angeles, CA 90048
(310) 838-6122, (800) 677-2368
The Michael Scholes School for Aromatic Studies is the only company in the United States that specializes in aromatherapy education. Its comprehensive program ranges from a two-day introduction to aromatherapy to a five-day certification course, with specialized programs for more advanced students. Interested people unable to attend the classes in person can use audio and video home study courses. In addition, Aromatherapy Seminars offers essential oils and aromatherapy products by mail order.

Aroma di Fioré
550 Center St., Ste. 113
Moraga, CA 94556
(510) 376-1108

Beginning and advanced classes and workshops. Also aromatherapy products, personal consultations, and a newsletter.

Lifetree Aromatix
3949 Longridge
Sherman Oaks, CA 91423
(818) 986-0594

Quintessence Aromatherapy
P.O. Box 4996
Boulder, CO 80306

Mindy Wilson, Aromatherapy Educator
5852 Richmond Ave.
Garden Grove, CA 92645
(714) 892-2386

Selected Bibliography

Bardeau, Fabrice. *La Medecine par les Fleurs*, 1976.

Belaiche, P., and M. Girault, Eds. *Traité de Phytotherapie et d'Aromatherapie*, Vol. 3. Paris: Maloine Editeur, 1979. Provides extensive clinical data. P. Belaiche teaches aromatherapy in French medical schools.

Cunningham, Scott. *Magical Aromatherapy*. St. Paul, MN: Llewellyn Publications, 1990. Explores different avenues for the uses of essential oils. Comprehensive and well written.

Davis, Patricia. *Aromatherapy: An A–Z*. Saffron Walden (Essex, England): C. W. Daniel, 1988. Patricia Davis founded the London School of Aromatherapy.

Franchomme, P., and D. Pénoél. *L'Aromathérapie exactement*. Limoges: Roger Jollois, 1990.

Gattefosse, R. M. *Aromatherapy*. Paris: Girardot, 1928. Gattefosse coined the term "aromatherapy."

Jackson, Judith. *Scentual Touch*. New York: Henry Holt, 1986.

Leclerc, H. *Précis de Phytotherapie*. Paris: Masson, 1954.

Maury, Marguerite. *The Secret of Life and Youth*, 1961. Once a collector's item, now available as *Mme. Maury's Guide to Aromatherapy*. Saffron Walden (Essex, England): C. W. Daniel, 1988.

Price, Shirley. *Practical Aromatherapy*. Rochester, VT: Thorsons Publishing Group, 1983.

Ryman, Danielle. *The Aromatherapy Handbook*. Saffron Walden (Essex, England): C. W. Daniel, 1984.

Tisserand, Robert. *The Art of Aromatherapy*. New York: Destiny Books, 1977. The British classic.

Tisserand, Robert. *Aromatherapy to Heal and Tend the Body*. Wilmot, WI: Lotus Light, 1989. Some interesting case studies.

Valnet, Jean. *The Practice of Aromatherapy*. Paris: Maloine, 1964 [American translation: Destiny Books, New York]. Still a classic, by the man who launched the revival of aromatherapy in France.

Valnet, J., C. Durrafour, and J. C. Lappraz. *Phytotherapie et Aromatherapie: Une medecine nouvelle*. Paris: Presses de la Renaissance, 1979. Drs. Durrafour and Lappraz also teach aromatherapy in France and Switzerland.

Worwood, Valerie. *Aromantics*. London: Pan Books, 1987. Funny, well written, provocative. Certainly a different perspective.

Worwood, Valerie. *The Complete Book of Essential Oils and Aromatherapy*. San Rafael, CA: New World Library, 1991.

Worwood, Valerie *The Fragrant Mind*. London: Doubleday, 1995.

ANTHROPOSOPHY

Goethe. *Metamorphose des plantes*. Paris: Editions Triades.

Gumbel, Dietrich. *Principles of Holistic Skin Therapy with Herbal Essences*. Heidelberg, Germany: Karl F. Haug Publishers, 1986.

Pelikan, Wilhelm. *Heilpflanzenkunde*, two volumes. Paris: Editions Triades, 1962. Absolutely fascinating. Explains in great detail the energy aspect of medicinal plants and the botanical

family approach. Available only in German and French.

ESSENTIAL OILS (PRODUCTION)

Arctander, Steffen. *Perfume and Flavor Materials of Natural Origin*. Self-published, 6665 Valley View Blvd., Las Vegas, NV 89118, 1960.

Guenther, E. *The Essential Oils*, Vol. 4, 1948–1952. Forty years later, still the bible. For serious, committed readers only (over 10,000 pages).

Lawrence, Brian. *Essential Oils, 1976–1978, 1979–1980, 1981–1987*, three volumes. Wheaton, Ill: Allured Publishing, Reprints from Dr. Lawrence's columns in "Perfumer & Flavorist." If Guenther is the bible, Lawrence could become the new testament. For experts only.

PERFUMERY, COSMETICS, AND FRAGRANCES

Gattefosse, R. M., and H. Jonquieres. *Techniques of Beauty Products*, 1949.

Genders, Roy. *A History of Scents*, 1972.

Gibbons, Boyd. "The Intimate Sense of Smell." *National Geographic*, Sept. 1986. Still a major landmark for the public awareness of the psychological effects of fragrances. Came with a very successful scratch and sniff test.

McKenzie, D. *Aromatics and the Soul*, 1923.

Miller, Richard and Iona. *The Magical and Ritual Use of Perfumes*, Rochester, VT: Inner Traditions, 1990.

Moncrieff, R.W. *Odors*, 1970.

Morris, Edwin T. *Fragrance: The Story of Perfume from Cleopatra to Chanel*. New York: Charles Scribner's Sons, 1984.

Poucher, William A. *Perfumes, Cosmetics and Soaps*, three volumes. Princeton: Van Nostrad, 1958.

Rimmel, E. *The Book of Perfumes*. London, 1865.

Thompson, C. J. S. *The Mystery and Lure of Perfumes*. Philadelphia: Lippincott, 1927.

Theimer, Ernst. *Fragrance Chemistry: The Science of the Sense of Smell*. Academic Press, San Diego, 1982.

Van Toller, Steve, and George Dodd, Eds. *Perfumery: The Psychology and Biology of Fragrance*. London/New York: Chapman & Hall, 1988. Conceived following the First International Conference on the Psychology of Perfumery. Fascinating. The authors conduct research at the University of Warwick in England.

TRADITION

Lemery, Nicholas. *Dictionaire des drogues simples*, 1759.

Braunschweig, Hieronymus. *The vertuose boke of distyllacyon of the waters of all maner of herbes*, 1527.

Mayer, Joseph E. *The Herbalist*, 1907.

PERIODICALS

The International Journal of Aromatherapy. Aromatherapy Publications, 3 Shirley Street, Hove, E. Sussex BN3 3WJ, England. Edited by Robert Tisserand; available through the AATA.

Perfumer and Flavorist. Allured Publishing Corporation, PO Box 318, Wheaton, IL 60189-0318, USA.

The Journal of Essential Oil Research. Allured Publishing Corporation, PO Box 318, Wheaton, IL 60189-0318, USA.

Index of
Essential Oils

bold denotes primary listing

Index

[handwritten notes in margin:]
febrifuge
sudorific
cicatrizant
antiphlogistic
aperitive
vermifuge
ascariasis (75)
oxyuriasis